Success in Academic Surgery

Series editors:

Lillian Kao
The University of Texas Health Science Centre
Houston, Texas
USA

Herbert Chen
Department of Surgery
University of Alabama at Birmingham
Alabama
USA

Herbert Chen • Lillian S. Kao
Editors

Success in Academic Surgery

Second Edition

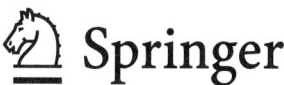

Editors
Herbert Chen, M.D.
Department of Surgery
University of Alabama at Birmingham
Birmingham, Alabama
USA

Lillian S. Kao, MD, M.S.
Department of Surgery
The University of Texas Health
Science Centre
Houston, TX
USA

ISSN 2194-7481 ISSN 2194-749X (electronic)
Success in Academic Surgery
ISBN 978-3-319-43951-8 ISBN 978-3-319-43952-5 (eBook)
DOI 10.1007/978-3-319-43952-5

Library of Congress Control Number: 2016959601

© Springer International Publishing Switzerland 2017
This work is subject to copyright. All rights are reserved by the Publisher, whether the whole or part of the material is concerned, specifically the rights of translation, reprinting, reuse of illustrations, recitation, broadcasting, reproduction on microfilms or in any other physical way, and transmission or information storage and retrieval, electronic adaptation, computer software, or by similar or dissimilar methodology now known or hereafter developed.
The use of general descriptive names, registered names, trademarks, service marks, etc. in this publication does not imply, even in the absence of a specific statement, that such names are exempt from the relevant protective laws and regulations and therefore free for general use.
The publisher, the authors and the editors are safe to assume that the advice and information in this book are believed to be true and accurate at the date of publication. Neither the publisher nor the authors or the editors give a warranty, express or implied, with respect to the material contained herein or for any errors or omissions that may have been made.

Printed on acid-free paper

This Springer imprint is published by Springer Nature
The registered company is Springer International Publishing AG Switzerland
The registered company is Gewerbestrasse 11, 6330 Cham, Switzerland

Foreword

With the first publication of *Success in Academic Surgery*, its introduction in 2012 inaugurated a highly readable, concisely written, forward-thinking, and progressive attempt to provide the imminent tools essential for maturation and development of an academic surgeon. The second edition of *Success in Academic Surgery* outlines a similar methodological approach in chapter formatting, length, and content with evolving state-of-the-art principles and tenets considered paramount to success for the aspiring young academic surgeon whose practice, research initiatives, and teaching will be principally in an Academic Medical Center (AMC).

These initiatives will require the academic surgeon as the "bridge-tender" so eloquently discussed in the last edition by Dr. Scott Lemaire. Parenthetically, the "bridge-tender" metaphor precisely depicts the critical and inspirational role expected of the academic teaching surgeon to "bridge" the developmental interface expected from the patient's bedside to bench-translational site, then back to bedside to initiate research application for patient care. Arguably, the best "bridge-tender" (a term inspired and attributed to Dr. Francis D. Moore of the Brigham Hospital) is required and as revered today as in the formative days of physicians' education within the Halstedian residency at Johns Hopkins University.

In the clinical scenario, the surgical scientist is increasingly challenged by the emphasis of academic evaluation and progress for accomplishing the three quintessential domains expected of all academic surgeons: clinician-*surgeon*, bench-translational *researcher*, and resident-student *teacher*. For the majority of AMCs in the United States and Canada, the Chair and Division Directors of Departments provide succinct, recurrent, evaluable data that will be processed as part of the individual academic surgeon's personnel files; these documents identify and define academic progress with requisite justification for promotion as a criteria of objective evaluation of his/her performance in these three areas of surgical academia. Faculty scholars have observed in virtually all Schools of Medicine within the AMC the evident chasm that exists for demands of academic advancement placed upon the time schedule, work effort, and career enhancement of the surgical scientist. Many forward-thinking surgical faculty attempt to balance their work and time allocation in the three daily modicums for progress and success. Early in the surgical scientist's career, a necessary link exists between observational sciences and prospectively designed clinical trials to provide insightful correlation with hypothesis-driven scientific query; thereafter, these evolving scientists share opinions/observations that drive laboratory experimentation with clinical translation followed by phase I-III clinical trials. Quite simply put, implementation of surgical science is essential to advance patient care, quality safety outcomes, and cost reduction in an unforgiving health care society of the twenty-first century in which the GDP of the United States for health care is the highest percentile (17.5%) of all industrialized societies in the world.

As a past-President of the Association for Academic Surgery (AAS) Council, it is particularly fulfilling to observe the culmination and achievement of the Association that has provided profound impact for the development and success of surgical scientists that were mentored by active and senior members of the Association. The success of the Council-directed AAS courses in fundamental research was inclusive of the AAS Fundamentals of Surgical Research (FSRC); this tome links its organization and success to past and present AAS Council and Membership who saw that advocacy of a rewarding academic surgical career was based upon the tenets put forth in this 2017 publication of the second edition. The mentoring and leadership required of these senior faculty members with their mentoring skills began with research themes: "How to Construct and Develop a Manuscript," "Methodologies of Research for the Projects Chosen," and "Hypothesis Development" and are considered attributes achieved by former nascent scientists and clinicians who became mentor-teachers and dedicated investigators themselves. Unequivocally, the most valued attribute of an academic surgical mentor is their "grit" to sustain and contribute to mentees in all disciplines of the surgical sciences. Moreover, this book is well balanced and teaches several techniques to become an outstanding mentor of young clinician-scientists, for example, how to write and obtain funding, methods to sustain research excellence following establishment of a successful laboratory in fundamental science, and ultimately, requisite measures to become an independent investigator. Additionally, time management and work-life balance are discussed, as they are paramount to both academic satisfaction and family development, both of which encourage a fulfilling and successful career with avoidance of "work burn-out."

With few exceptions, all nascent young scientists and surgery students/residents who desire an academic career will typically formulate these decisions based upon prior interaction with a revered and supportive mentor. Coined by Homer in his classic epic, *The Odyssey*, the "mentor" is a trusted friend who assumes responsibility for raising (teaching with accountability) the mentee. The mentoring achieved was directed to Odysseus' son, Telemachus, and delivered success and enablement of the son in Odysseus' absence. Thus, if we fast-forward the concept into contemporary academic surgery, the valued principle of mentoring is sustained and still operative in the twenty-first century to achieve highly regarded academic success in surgical science. First and foremost, the role of the mentor is that of a teacher, an advocate, and a critic. But, he or she as a mentor is expected to become the ultimate role model for the individual who chooses the laboratory or clinical service in which the mentee wishes to base their principle career aspirations. Thereafter, the mentor becomes their advocate, their advisor, their consultant, and the ultimate judge of their academic progress. Honesty is essential to be a successful mentor and to provide the mentee positive (and negative) outcomes of their progress to accurately amplify their talents and research prowess. With advisement of the mentor on development of an academic career, the mentee must have access to extensive knowledge of the variance and depth for methods of scholarly pursuit, participation and activity in professional activities, research administrative management, and evaluation of outcomes.

The authors of *Success in Academic Surgery (Second Edition)* have built upon the essential components described above regarding mentorship and its movement to the clinic, the laboratory, and the teaching wards. Typically, the nascent young academic launches their career with the highest expectations of achieving considerable success in all three domains of surgical academia. This daunting task and its variance are considerable, and some trainees do *not* wish to maintain or establish careers with full commitment to all domains of surgical science leadership. That said, the great majority of these young academics identify a niche in their career in which they are highly focused and experience meaningful success in one of the three areas. The opportunity to develop success in each of the principle domains of academics often portends a surgical leadership designation at subsequent dates. *Without exception, the greatest reward for the mentor is their ability to recruit, retain, and oversee development of successful academic careers of their chosen mentee.* The judgment of academic success resides principally in two areas: (1) success and proficiency in the clinical arena for various surgical disciplines, and (2) high-impact research publications and grants that answer critical scientific hypotheses with intent to enhance society through health care and survival improvement in these disciplines. Without question, the characteristic of the *ideal mentor* is an individual with demonstrative leadership skills that provide judgmental development of the mentee with empathy, inspiration, charismatic motivational skills, and generosity. As stated by L.A. Ladoz in 1986, effective teaching and mentoring is based upon "Mentors are guides"… "They lead us along the journey of our lives and we trust (mentors) because they have been here before. The mentor embodies our hopes, casts light on the way ahead, interprets arcane signs, warns us of dangers, and points out unexpected delights along the way." This statement pertains today as *the performance of the mentor is consistently judged by the success of the mentee*!

Drs. Chen and Kao have organized the second edition to strengthen requisite academic performance for the evolving, nascent surgical scientist to achieve success that can be sustained throughout their academic career. This second edition encourages and emphasizes the requirement of publications, awards, academic visibility, conference attendance, citizenship, and successful grant funding to achieve the ultimate accolade of success with national and international recognition as a surgical scientist. The many caveats of success are built upon determination, which is a requisite precept for principles espoused in this text to assist organizational development for the successful young scientist and clinician.

This edition provides guidance for all academicians on their focused paths for achievements in academic surgery. As was evident in the first edition, the authors recognize the dedication of the AAS as an entry-level academic surgical society that encourages and embellishes scientific accomplishment, structured principles of research, and advancement of knowledge to provide the necessary academic tools for success. All mentors and faculty colleagues agree that there is great promise of success for the aspiring clinician-scientist whose daily task focuses upon patient care, research, and teaching. The dedication of the multiple authors of the second edition of *Success in Academic Surgery* to achieve this objective is evident in the chapters that follow and form the basis of your mentorship for academic development.

Kirby I. Bland, M.D.
AAS Past-President, 1988
Professor, Division of Surgical Oncology
Chair *Emeritus,* UAB Department of Surgery
Distinguished Faculty Scholar, UAB School of Medicine
Senior Advisor, UAB Comprehensive Cancer Center

Preface

We are excited to serve as the Editors for the 2nd Edition of "Success in Academic Surgery." The first and second editions are based upon the Fundamentals of Surgical Research and the Career Development Courses taught by members of the Association for Academic Surgery (AAS). As Past Presidents of the AAS, we are very aware of the important contributions that the Association has made to fostering and mentoring generations of surgeons as they navigate the complex waters of academic surgery. Therefore, this book serves as a brief summary of the experiences and advice of several successful academic surgeons.

In addition to this book, we have established a series of texts which provide more details in specialized areas in academic surgery. These books include:

Leadership in Surgery, Editors: Melina R. Kibbe and Herbert Chen

Academic Global Surgery, Editors: Mamta Swaroop, Sanjay Krishnaswami

Success in Academic Surgery: Developing a Career in Surgical Education, Editors: Carla M. Pugh, Rebecca S. Sippel

Success in Academic Surgery: Basic Science, Editors: Melina R. Kibbe and Scott A LeMaire

Success in Academic Surgery: Clinical Trials, Editors: Timothy M. Pawlik and Julie A. Sosa

Success in Academic Surgery: Health Services Research, Editors Justin B. Dimick and Caprice C. Greenberg

Success in Academic Surgery: Surgical Quality Improvement, Editors Rachel R. Kelz and Sandra L. Wong

Success in Academic Surgery: A How To Guide for Medical Students, Editors Michael J. Englesbe and Michael O. Meyers

We would like to thank the authors and editors, all of whom have served in leadership roles within the AAS, for their time and efforts. We hope that these books will inspire the next generation of academic surgeons.

Houston, TX, USA Lillian S. Kao, M.D., M.S.
Birmingham, Alabama, USA Herbert Chen, M.D.

Contributor Current and Past Positions: Association for Academic Surgery

Daniel Albo, M.D., Ph.D.
President (2010–2011); Nominating Committee Chair (2010–2011); Recorder (2007–2009); Program Committee Chair (2007–2009); Councilor (2006–2008); Program Committee Member (2003–2006)

Malcolm V. Brock, M.D.
AAS Representative to the Society of Black Academic Surgeons (2008–2011)

F. Charles Brunicardi, M.D.
President (1997–1998); (1996–1997); Recorder (1994–1996); Chairman Program Committee, Association for Academic Surgery (1994–1996); Chairman Committee on Issues, Association for Academic Surgery (1993–1994); Committee on Issues (1992–1993)

Herbert Chen, M.D.
President (2008–2009); Nominating Committee Chair (2008–2009); Communications Committee (2005–2007); Recorder (2004–2007); Institutional Representative (2004–2007); Program Committee Chair (2004–2007); Committee on Leadership (2003–2006); Education Committee (2002–2004); Membership Committee (2000–2002); Audit Committee (2000–2001)

Justin B. Dimick, M.D., M.P.H
President (2015–2016); Secretary (2012–2014); Chair, Outcomes Research Committee (2011–2013); AAS Representative to the Surgical Outcomes Club (2010–2011)

David P. Foley, M.D.
AAS Representative to the National Association for Biomedical Research (2011–2013); Co-Chair Education Committee (2010–2011); Education Committee (2009–2011)

Steven B. Goldin, M.D., Ph.D.
Co-Director of the Fundamentals of Surgical Research Course (2010–2011); Education Committee (2009–2011)

Caprice C. Greenberg, M.D., M.P.H
President (2016–2017); Recorder (2013–2015); AAS Representative to the Surgical Outcomes Club (2011–2013)

Andrea A. Hayes-Jordan, M.D.
Ethics Committee Chair (2011–2013); AAS Representative to the American College of Surgeons Board of Governors (2010–2011)

Lillian S. Kao, M.D., M.S.
President (2013–2014); Secretary (2010–2012); AAS/Royal Australasian College of Surgeons Task Force (2010–2012 [Chair]); AAS Foundation Board of Directors (2010–2012); Co-Chair Leadership Committee (2009–2010); Co-Chair Education Committee (2008–2009); Institutional Representative (2007–2010); Education Committee Member (2007–2008)

Melina R. Kibbe, M.D., RVT
President (2012–2013); Recorder (2009–2011); Program Committee Chair (2009–2011); IT Committee (2008); Issues Committee Chair (2007–2008); Issues Committee Member (2006–2008); Institutional Representative (2005–2007)

Scott A. LeMaire, M.D.
President (2011–2012); Secretary (2008–2010); Academic Surgical Congress Core Committee (2010–2012); AAS/Royal Australasian College of Surgeons Course Task Force (2009–2010 [Chair]); AAS Foundation Board of Directors (2008–2010, 2011–2012); Leadership Committee (2006–2008 [Co-Chair, 2007–2008]); Committee on Issues (2004–2006 [Chair, 2005–2006]); Program Committee (2001–2003)

Peter R. Nelson, M.D., M.S.
Chair, Program Committee (2011–2013); Nominating Committee (2009–2010); Co-Chair, Leadership Committee (2008–2010); Co-Chair, AAS Career Development Course (2008–2010); AAS Visiting Professor, Younger Fellows, Royal Australasian College of Surgeons (2009); Chair, Membership Committee (2006–2008); Membership Committee (2003–2006); Institutional Representative (2005–2007)

Fiemu E. Nwariaku, M.D.
President (2007–2008)

Timothy M. Pawlik, M.D., M.P.H
President (2014–2015); Treasurer (2010–2013); Deputy Treasurer (2009–2010); Councilor (2007–2009)

Carla M. Pugh, M.D., Ph.D.
Councilor (2010–2012); Nominating Committee Member (2009–2010); Education Committee Co-Chair (2008–2009); Education Committee Member (2007–2008)

Taylor S. Riall, M.D., Ph.D.
Councilor (2009–2011); Membership Committee (2008–2009); AAS Program Committee (2007–2008)

C. Max Schmidt, M.D., Ph.D., MBA
AAS Treasurer (2007–2010); AAS Foundation Secretary-Treasurer (2010–2011); Coordinator, AAS French College of Surgeons Inaugural Course (2009–2011); AAS-SUS Conflict of Interest Committee (2009–2010); AAS Foundation (2007–2011); Chair, AAS Audit Committee (2007–2010); AAS Institutional Representative (2007–2010); AAS Program Committee (2006–2007); AAS Committee on Issues (2002–2004)

Margaret L. Schwarze, M.D.
Ethics Committee Chair (2009–2011)

Julie Ann Sosa, M.A., M.D.
AAS Recorder (2011–2013); AAS Representative to the American College of Surgeons Surgical Research Committee (2009–2011)

Christoph Troppmann, M.D.
Councilor (2010–2012); Program Committee (2008–2010); Committee on Issues (2006–2008); AAS Program Committee (2003–2006)

Kathrin Troppmann, M.D.
Deputy Treasurer (2008–2009); Education Committee (2001–2003 [Chair, 2002–2003]); AAS Representative to the AAMC/Council of Academic Societies (2003–2009); Leadership Committee (2002–2003); Nominating Committee (2002–2003)

Contents

Part I Introduction

1 **Why Be an Academic Surgeon? Impetus and Options for the Emerging Surgeon-Scientist** 3
Scott A. LeMaire

2 **Timeline for Promotion/Overview of an Academic Career**........... 9
Peter R. Nelson

Part II Research: From Conception to Publication

3 **Reviewing the Literature, Developing a Hypothesis, Study Design** 25
Rosalie Carr and C. Max Schmidt

4 **Ethics in Surgical Research** 33
Richard A. Burkhart and Timothy M. Pawlik

5 **Study Design and Analysis in Clinical Research** 47
Hemalkumar B. Mehta and Taylor S. Riall

6 **Animal Models for Surgical Research** 69
Andrea A. Hayes-Jordan

7 **Health Services Research** 79
Caprice C. Greenberg and Justin B. Dimick

8 **Surgical Educational Research: Getting Started** 95
Roger H. Kim

9 **Translational Research and New Approaches: Genomics, Proteomics, and Metabolomics** 107
David P. Foley

| 10 | How to Write and Revise a Manuscript for Peer Review Publication.................................. | 119 |

Melina R. Kibbe

Part III Critical Elements for Success

| 11 | Choosing, and Being, a Good Mentor......................... | 135 |

Tracy S. Wang and Julie Ann Sosa

| 12 | Writing a Grant/Obtaining Funding.......................... | 145 |

Aaron J. Dawes and Melinda Maggard-Gibbons

| 13 | Setting Up a 'Lab' (Clinical or Basic Science Research Program) and Managing a Research Team.............................. | 161 |

Fiemu E. Nwariaku

Part IV Work-Life Balance

| 14 | Work-Life Balance and Burnout............................. | 175 |

Kathrin M. Troppmann and Christoph Troppmann

| 15 | Time Management .... | 187 |

Carla M. Pugh and Jay N. Nathwani

Index... 201

Contributors

Malcolm V. Brock, M.D. Department of Surgery and Oncology, Johns Hopkins School of Medicine, Baltimore, MD, USA

Department of Environmental Health Sciences, Johns Hopkins Bloomberg School of Public Health, Baltimore, MD, USA

Richard A. Burkhart, M.D. Department of Surgery, Johns Hopkins University School of Medicine, Baltimore, MD, USA

Rosalie Carr, MD Department of Surgery, Department of Biochemistry and Molecular Biology, Indiana University School of Medicine, Indianapolis, IN, USA

Aaron J. Dawes, M.D., Ph.D. Department of Surgery, David Geffen School of Medicine at UCLA, Los Angeles, CA, USA

Justin B. Dimick, M.D., M.P.H. Department of Surgery, Center for Healthcare Outcomes and Policy, University of Michigan, Ann Arbor, MI, USA

David P. Foley, M.D. Department of Surgery, Division of Organ Transplantation, University of Wisconsin School of Medicine and Public Health, Madison, WI, USA

Caprice C. Greenberg, M.D., M.P.H. Department of Surgery, University of Wisconsin Hospitals and Clinics, Madison, WI, USA

Andrea A. Hayes-Jordan, M.D. Department of Surgical Oncology, UT MD Anderson Cancer Center, Houston, TX, USA

Melina R. Kibbe, M.D., RVT Department of Surgery, University of North Carolina, Chapel Hill, NC, USA

Roger H. Kim, MD Louisiana State University Health Sciences Center – Shreveport, Shreveport, LA, USA

Scott A. LeMaire, M.D. Division of Cardiothoracic Surgery, Michael E. DeBakey Department of Surgery, Baylor College of Medicine, Texas Heart Institute at St. Luke's Episcopal Hospital, Houston, TX, USA

Melinda Maggard-Gibbons, M.D., M.S.H.S. UCLA Medical Center, Department of Surgery, Los Angeles, CA, USA

Hemalkumar B. Mehta, Ph.D. Department of Surgery, University of Texas Medical Branch, Galveston, TX, USA

Jay N. Nathwani Department of Surgery, University of Wisconsin-Madison, School of Medicine and Public Health, Madison, WI, USA

Peter R. Nelson, M.D., M.S. Department of Surgery, Division of Vascular Surgery, University of Florida College of Medicine, Gainesville, FL, USA

Fiemu E. Nwariaku, M.D. Department of Surgery, University of Texas Southwestern Medical School, Dallas, TX, USA

Timothy M. Pawlik, M.D., M.P.H. Department of Surgery, The Ohio State University Wexner Medical Center, Columbus, OH, USA

Carla M. Pugh, M.D., Ph.D. Department of Surgery, University of Wisconsin-Madison, School of Medicine and Public Health, Madison, WI, USA

Taylor S. Riall, M.D., Ph.D. Department of Surgery, University of Arizona, Tucson, AZ, USA

C. Max Schmidt, M.D., Ph.D., MBA Department of Surgery, Department of Biochemistry and Molecular Biology, Indiana University School of Medicine, Indianapolis, IN, USA

Julie Ann Sosa, M.A., M.D., F.A.C.S. Section of Endocrine Surgery, Surgical Center for Outcomes Research (SCORES), Endocrine Neoplasia Diseases Group, Duke Cancer Institute and Duke Clinical Research Institute, Duke University, DUMC #2945, Durham, NC, USA

Christoph Troppmann, M.D. Department of Surgery, University of California, Davis, Sacramento, CA, USA

Kathrin Troppmann, M.D. Department of Surgery, University of California, Davis, Sacramento, CA, USA

Tracy S. Wang, M.D., M.P.H., F.A.C.S. Division of Surgical Oncology, Section of Endocrine Surgery, Medical College of Wisconsin, Milwaukee, WI, USA

Part I
Introduction

Chapter 1
Why Be an Academic Surgeon? Impetus and Options for the Emerging Surgeon-Scientist

Scott A. LeMaire

I cannot imagine a career more rewarding than that of an academic surgeon. This is the simple message I attempt to impart when mentoring students and trainees considering a career as a surgical scientist. The conversations that ensue in response to this proclamation invariably delve into the overarching questions of "What?", "Why?", and "How?" Although most of this book will guide you in the "How", in this brief introduction I will focus on the "What" and the "Why" by defining the academic surgeon, describing the enormous impact academic surgeons have on the world, and providing examples of the various types of surgical research that can lead to fulfilling academic careers.

Academic Surgeons as Bridge-Tenders

The simplest and most elegant definition of the academic surgeon I have encountered is attributed to the legendary surgeon-scientist, Dr. Francis D. Moore. In Dr. Graham Hill's account of his own early experiences that inspired him to become an academic surgeon, he focused on his brief exposure to the icon during Dr. Moore's visiting professorship at Otago Medical School in Dunedin, New Zealand. Dr. Hill recounted that Dr. Moore "saw himself as a 'bridge-tender', shuttling ideas, information, and discoveries between the bedside and the laboratory." Further, Dr. Moore "regarded being a surgeon-scientist as both a 'miracle and a privilege'. He inspired me, a young surgeon-in-training, to commit to academic surgery as the main interest of my professional life."

S.A. LeMaire, M.D.
Michael E. DeBakey Department of Surgery, Baylor College of Medicine, One Baylor Plaza, BCM 390, Houston, TX 77030, USA

Department of Cardiovascular Surgery, The Texas Heart Institute, Houston, TX, USA

© Springer International Publishing Switzerland 2017
H. Chen, L.S. Kao (eds.), *Success in Academic Surgery*,
Success in Academic Surgery, DOI 10.1007/978-3-319-43952-5_1

The bridge-tender metaphor is both apropos and inspirational. It positions the academic surgeon as the critical link between the patient's bedside and the proverbial laboratory bench. The process starts with a question that arises from dissatisfaction with the status quo: "How can we do better for our patients?" Clinical observations—whether in the emergency center, operating room, intensive care unit, clinic, hospital ward, or community—lead the surgeon-scientist to ask such questions and formulate hypotheses. These hypotheses are then brought directly to the "bench"—which can take the form of a molecular biology laboratory, an animal laboratory, a clinical venue, a database, or even a training program—where relevant experiments are performed with dogged tenacity. The ultimate goal is to bring the knowledge gained back to the clinical arena, with resulting improvements in patient care.

As Dr. Ray Chiu eloquently argued, such bridge tenders are needed more today than ever before. The increasing complexity of both clinical medicine and basic science has created a gulf between the two disciplines that "is getting deeper and wider." As the chasm continues to expand, the role of the surgeon-scientist becomes increasingly crucial in ensuring that research is driven by important clinical questions and that scientific discoveries are effectively applied to patient care. State-of-the art science simply cannot improve patient care without a direct link between the bench and bedside; academic surgeons provide that essential connection.

The "Impact Factor" of the Academic Surgeon

The **impact factor** is a measurement used by scientific journals to evaluate their relative importance within their field. In a similar manner, surgeons should consider their own impact factor by asking, "What impact will I have on the care of patients now and in the future?"

As surgeons, we have a unique opportunity to care for our patients by using both our intellect and our hands. The clinical impact of surgical care is enormous. We touch patients' lives by enabling them to live longer and with better quality of life (Fig. 1.1a).

Academic surgeons, of course, also have direct clinical impact through patient care, but they do much, much more (Fig. 1.1b). First, they have a scientific impact by conducting research that advances their field. Advances in surgical science ultimately influence patient care, greatly amplifying the academic surgeon's opportunity to improve patients' lives. Countless scientific advances led by surgeons—including hyperalimentation, cardiopulmonary bypass, organ transplantation, mechanical circulatory support, joint replacement, and synthetic vascular grafts—continue to benefit millions of patients every year. The clinical impact of surgeon-scientists is truly immeasurable.

Next, through teaching, academic surgeons impart knowledge and skills to the next generation of surgeons. Through clinical teaching, surgeons train students and trainees to develop the necessary cognitive and technical skills required to effectively

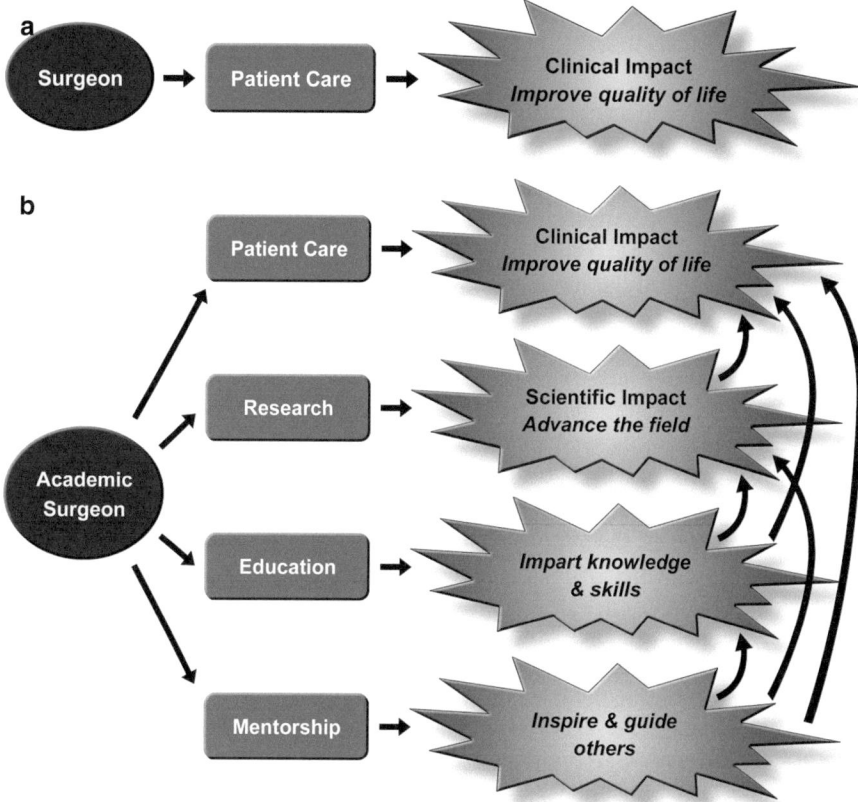

Fig. 1.1 (**a**) Surgeons have a tremendous impact on the lives of their patients. (**b**) For academic surgeons, this impact is amplified immeasurably through research, education, and mentorship

diagnose and treat surgical disease. Academic surgeons enjoy the additional privilege of teaching future scientists as they learn the many skills necessary to conduct and communicate research, such as by critically evaluating the literature, developing a pertinent hypothesis, planning suitable experiments, performing appropriate statistical analyses, writing effective abstracts, manuscripts, and grant proposals, and giving cogent presentations. Trainees go on to use this knowledge in their scientific and clinical careers, further expanding the overall impact the academic surgeon has on the world.

Finally, through mentorship, academic surgeons inspire and guide others in achieving their goals. No one achieves success in medicine and science without the encouragement, counsel, and selfless support of a group of mentors. Serving in this capacity for others and helping them realize their dreams enables us to pay it forward and is immensely rewarding. As mentees develop their own careers, we share in their clinical, scientific, and educational accomplishments.

Types of Surgical Research

There are several major categories of surgical research to choose from as one embarks on a career in academic surgery. As described in detail in subsequent chapters, each type of research requires a specific set of skills beyond those acquired during clinical training. In **basic science research**, the investigator performs laboratory experiments to answer fundamental biological questions that are relevant to surgical care. The central themes of surgical basic science research generally include the molecular and cellular mechanisms that cause disease, and biological responses to injury, disease, and surgical treatment. Examples of basic science research projects include investigating immune responses to trauma and hemorrhage by using an animal model, performing experiments with transgenic mice to determine whether the absence of a gene prevents tumor metastasis, and using cell cultures to find out whether a drug prevents cytokine release in response to oxidative stress.

In **translational research**, the investigator focuses on directly linking laboratory discoveries and clinical care. This type of research perhaps best exemplifies the bridge-tender role of the surgeon-scientist. The potential clinical significance of translational research is distinctly palpable and serves as an ever-present source of motivation. Examples of translational research projects include evaluating human vein graft samples with microarrays to determine whether a specific expression profile predicts graft failure, identifying diagnostic biomarkers for human hepatocellular carcinoma by using mass spectrometry, and determining whether administration of a new drug reduces protease expression in human aortic aneurysm tissue.

Clinical studies answer questions about surgical diseases and treatments by using human subjects. Clinical research varies substantially in scope and complexity. Retrospective studies involving well-defined cohorts of patients can provide important information that can be used to characterize the status quo and generate hypotheses. Prospective clinical studies enable surgeons to further refine our understanding of the clinical history of disease and the outcomes of various forms of treatment. The jewel in the crown of clinical research is the randomized clinical trial. Like clinical research in general, clinical trials exhibit considerable diversity. Examples of clinical trials include a single-center trial to determine whether cerebrospinal fluid drainage during aortic repair prevents spinal cord complications, a multicenter trial to compare the outcomes of laparoscopic-assisted resection vs. open resection of rectal cancer, and an industry-sponsored, multicenter trial to evaluate the safety and efficacy of a new sealant developed to prevent anastomotic leaks.

Outcomes research, also called **health services research**, seeks to reveal the end results of specific health care practices and interventions. This area of research utilizes advanced epidemiologic techniques to link social and process issues—such as ethnic disparities in health care access, low procedural volume, trainee work-hour restrictions, and the introduction of safety initiatives—with clinical and financial outcomes such as survival, quality of life, and hospital costs. The popularity of outcomes research has necessarily increased over the past few years in parallel with the medical profession's expanding focus on health care policy, evidence-based practice guidelines, patient safety, and resource allocation. Examples of outcomes research include determining whether surgical mortality is related to hospital volume by using a national database, evaluating the long-term impact of bariatric procedures through longitudinal measurement of quality of life, and determining whether ethnicity correlates with graft failure and survival after liver transplantation by using United Network for Organ Sharing registry data.

Surgical education research seeks to understand the factors that affect surgical training. Recent challenges to longstanding training paradigms have created a pressing need to improve our approach to surgical education. Surgical educators need to efficiently train surgeons to perform increasingly complex procedures in a manner that optimizes both patient safety and resource utilization while meeting expanding regulations related to work hours; much of surgical education research is directed specifically at developing and validating methods to accomplish this goal. Examples of surgical education research include comparing the effectiveness of computer-aided simulation vs. animal lab training for teaching advanced laparoscopic procedures, evaluating the effects of teaching techniques on trainee retention of lecture material, and determining whether medical students with the best technical skills choose careers in surgical specialties.

Going Forward

In summary, choosing a career in academic surgery enables one to provide state-of-the-art clinical care, discover and apply new knowledge to surgical problems, teach trainees and surgeons throughout the world, and inspire others toward ever-greater achievements. Each type of surgical research—basic science, translational, clinical, outcomes, and education—enables surgeon-scientists to advance the field and amplify their impact on patients' lives.

Having addressed the "What" and the "Why", the remainder of this book will focus on how to become a successful academic surgeon. As you move forward, I encourage you to periodically reflect on what your impact factor will be and to keep in mind one simple message: there is no career more rewarding than that of an academic surgeon.

Acknowledgments The author wishes to thank Stephen N. Palmer, PhD, ELS, for editorial assistance, and Scott A. Weldon, MA, CMI, for assistance with the illustrations.

Selected Reading

1. Chiu RC. The challenge of "tending the bridge". Ann Thorac Surg. 2008;85:1149–50.
2. Cosimi AB. Surgeons and the Nobel Prize. Arch Surg. 2006;141:340–8.
3. Hill GL. Surgeon scientist: adventures in surgical research. Auckland: Random House New Zealand; 2006.
4. Moore FD. A miracle and a privilege: recounting a half century of surgical advance. Washington, DC: Joseph Henry Press; 1995.
5. Murphy AM, Cameron DE. The Blalock-Taussig-Thomas collaboration: a model for medical progress. JAMA. 2008;300:328–30.

Chapter 2
Timeline for Promotion/Overview of an Academic Career

Peter R. Nelson

Introduction

Promotion simply defined focuses on (1) the concept of advancement, but more broadly includes (2) the encouragement of progress, growth, or acceptance of something, and (3) advertisement for that advancement. This three-tiered definition is consistent with the concept of promotion in the realm of academic surgery. For us, promotion is not only the primary metric of recognition for professional advancement, but also the very enticement for the hard work and accomplishment along the way. Ultimately, the advertisement or publicity comes with the use of your professional title on your CV, your business cards, and in other business interactions within the medical field. Promotion, by way of advancement of this professional title from instructor to assistant professor, to associate professor, and eventually to full professor, then serves as the gauge of progress along the time continuum that makes up one's academic surgical career (Fig. 2.1).

Seen in that light, promotion is therefore a critically important concept, yet one for which there is generally no formal teaching and one that is arguably poorly conveyed through your formative years of medical school and residency. How, therefore, are we supposed to navigate the process without any guidance or experience? This chapter is designed to get you started, to provide the basic concepts and a basic framework. It comes less from textbooks or the literature, but largely from the author's experiences and those of his peers' through lectures delivered at the Association for Academic Surgery's Fundamentals of Surgical Research and Career Development Courses. However, at the end you will find a brief bibliography that will direct you to additional material on the subject.

P.R. Nelson
Department of Surgery, Division of Vascular Surgery, University of Florida College of Medicine, Gainesville, FL, USA

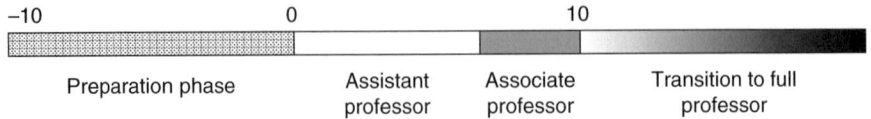

Fig. 2.1 Overall promotion timeline

Preparation Phase

If you look at Fig. 2.2, it spans roughly a 20-year period over which you need to acquire the credentials upon which you will be judged for promotion. So this takes foresight and preemptive planning, even well before your first faculty appointment. Many of the readers may already be in their first academic job, and as such, may have missed the opportunity to orchestrate this planning phase, but I am guessing many of you accomplished this phase, either consciously or subconsciously, to get to your current position.

The process really begins in undergraduate school, or at the very least, in the preclinical years of medical school. Somewhere along the line you must have been exposed to research to a sufficient degree that this experience, or perhaps an individual person with whom you worked, influenced your decision to pursue an academic career in medicine. You may have done research as a summer National Research Service Award (NRSA) scholar as an undergraduate, or you may have decided to go on to graduate school to pursue a full PhD. Others may have decided to pursue a combined MD-PhD degree, while still others may have just done research along the way in an advanced scholar's track that promoted research and academics. Whichever path you took, it is here that you first learned the importance of a good research idea or question, were introduced to the scientific method used to investigate and analyze that question, and perhaps were even given the opportunity to present and publish your findings. These concepts and experiences provide the critical tools upon which to build your initial academic skill set.

The next step in this preparation phase is the selection of an academic residency program in which to train. You need to seek out a program that will not only train you well clinically, but one that maintains a strong commitment to academics and provides resources for residents to spend dedicated time doing research. Research fellowships offered by the National Institutes of Health (NIH) (i.e., T32 training grants) generally supply a resident with 2 years of salary and research funding and are one of the best support mechanisms for this activity (Table 2.1). Traditionally, funding was intended for residents in a basic science lab of a surgical mentor doing conventional bench-top research, but more recently, training programs and opportunities have expanded to include similar support for translational research, clinical research, health sciences (outcomes) research, and/or education-based research. Other institution-based NIH-training programs are often available for these additional pursuits such as a K30- program that provides tuition for additional course-

2 Timeline for Promotion/Overview of an Academic Career   11

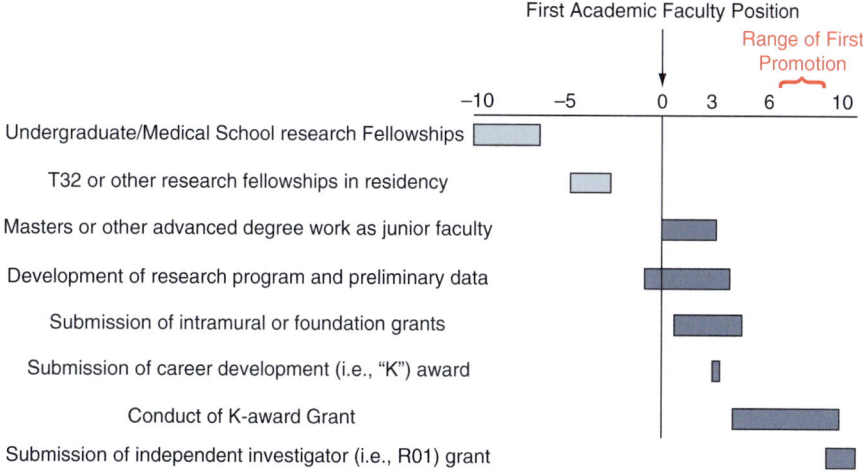

Fig. 2.2 Detailed timeline to first promotion

Table 2.1 Select NIH program offerings that support resident academic training

NIH mechanism	Description
T32	Ruth L. Kirschstein National Research Service Award (NRSA) Institutional Research Training Grants
K12	Academic Development Award
K30	Clinical Research Curriculum Award
F30	Ruth L. Kirschstein National Research Service Awards for Individual Predoctoral MD/PhD and Other Dual Doctoral Degree Fellows
F31	Ruth L. Kirschstein National Research Service Awards for Individual Predoctoral Fellows
F32	Ruth L. Kirschstein National Research Service Awards (NRSA) for Individual Postdoctoral Fellows

Adapted from National Institutes of Health (http://grants.nih.gov/grants/guide/parent_announcements.htm)

work or a K12-program that provides salary support to cover time away from clinical activity (Table 2.1). These programs often offer the opportunity to complete a Master's degree in public health (MPH) or with a concentration in clinical research. For the dedicated resident, many programs will collaborate with the graduate school to offer the opportunity to spend a third dedicated research year to complete a full PhD. For still others with unique interests, time and support might be provided to pursue law or business administration degrees if applicable. The key point however is that, although some research can be done along the way without dedicated time, a focused commitment, independent of the field of research, is really essential for the acquisition of the basic skills needed to eventually be tooled to establish a research program and successfully compete for independent funding.

Assistant Professor

Job Search

The next critical step in your academic career is the review and selection of your first academic faculty appointment. This may be singularly the most important step toward success in academic surgery, because you are the primary driving force for that success, but you need the right environment in which to thrive. As you evaluate opportunities, you need to carefully examine the people in the department and division you will be joining. Are they good people? Have they been successful and achieved promotion? Is their academic career stable enough that they will be willing to make your development a priority? These are all important questions that can be difficult to determine in a couple of recruitment visits, but you need to get the best sense of it that you can.

Other than those overriding questions, what sorts of things should you specifically negotiate for? One of the most popular items on the recruitee's list is often the concept of "protected time." It is common for people to recommend that you request 50% protected time for academic pursuits, and many jobs will be willing to include that in their offer (I even looked at a job that offered 100% protected time). However, someone once told me that "you need to protect yourself from yourself," meaning that we can at times be our own worst enemies. By always taking on that extra consult or OR case, an appointment to a committee or departmental project, or writing another chapter or review paper, we eat right into our own protected time. You need to have discipline early to be able to say "no" and respectfully decline opportunities that will distract you from your main objectives. Two points to make here: (1) the best situation for protected time is that your partners understand your mission and share your vision such that they don't make you feel bad or that "you owe them one" if they take care of something for you during academic time; and (2) if you get commitment for protected time, you better take advantage of it and use it wisely.

More important than protected time are the resources you ask/look for to support your academic pursuits. In addition to time, you will need space, money, and a research staff. You should try to get a committed research lab or space that is 600 sq. ft. in size or better and ideally all yours, but in and around other productive labs. This may be space in a larger open lab concept with your mentor for example, but should be your space to control. Where the space is located depends a little bit on you. If it's across from your clinical office, then you may never completely separate clinical and research activities because someone is always dropping in with clinical questions. On the other hand, if it is remote from your office, say in another building, then you will get separation, but at the expense of the convenience of dropping into the lab between cases. You have to decide. Next, seed money to get you started before you have a chance to submit grant applications is essential to generate preliminary data and get your program off the ground. An amount of $50,000 per year for 3–5 years is reasonable, but the more, the better. If you can get a $500,000 endowment for the lab, take it! Finally, research staff is critical. You may need to set up a small but efficient and productive team to get started. You should get a separate commitment for salary support for a lab technician, research nurse, or study coordinator depending on your needs, because these salaries are what will otherwise eat into your seed money quickly.

Equally, if not more important than these essential resources, assessing the availability of mentorship at your new institution is critical. Again, this can be hard during brief recruitment visits, so do your homework. Get on the university Web site and search for researchers working in areas of interest to you. Look up their publications on PubMed and their current funding in the NIH CRISP database. Then, specifically request to get them on your interview schedule so you can "interview" them as a potential mentor. There is an entire chapter dedicated to mentorship, but the essential things you need to identify in a potential mentor are their enthusiasm to help you, their availability in terms of not being overcommitted already, their available resources and core facilities, and their, and the department's, track-record of success in developing academic junior faculty. Having a head start identifying a mentor at this stage will be very beneficial to hitting the road running as soon as you arrive.

Finally, there are a few other things to pay attention to as you assess your first academic position. One is the state of the group's clinical practice. From your perspective, does the group have sufficient volume in your specific area of interest such that you can build an appealing clinical practice? Furthermore, does this clinical volume coincide with your area of research interest? If the answers to these questions are "yes," then it may be a good fit. On the other hand, do the existing partners seem overwhelmed with clinical work? Are they primarily looking for a new partner to contribute clinical activity (to decompress their own volume or to boost divisional work relative value units (RVU) or clinical revenue)? What is the departmental priority – clinical revenue or a balance of clinical and academic missions? And how is your salary supported – completely by clinical dollars, or in part by development money set aside for academic support? These latter questions are important because the answers will give you insight into whether you will truly have time and support for academic activities. A related concept to explore is the availability of a full- or part-time Veteran's Administration (VA) appointment. If the institution has an affiliated VA Hospital that the group staffs, then this is a nice place for a new junior faculty to get started. There is generally ample clinical volume, but usually not overwhelming, and is often very controllable and not tied to a strict RVU system. Therefore, organizing your time in the VA is much more conducive to defining and protecting research or academic time.

The First Three Years

Once you have settled on your first academic appointment, usually as an Assistant Professor, then it is time to immediately start thinking about what it will take for promotion. Figure 2.2 outlines one possible path to your first promotion; however, realize there are potentially many ways to get there. Also, the criteria and process for promotion vary widely from institution to institution, so it is critically important that you familiarize yourself with the process at your institution. In general, promotion is awarded for superior achievement in at least two of the following areas: patient care, teaching, research, and service. These areas of concentration may be differentially represented in different tracks that lead to promotion, and again there is significant variability here (Table 2.2). In surgery, excellence in patient care is a primary and consistent requirement; on the other hand, a service focus is rarely applicable. Therefore, the remainder is focused on either research or educational activities, or both. It is imperative that you understand your job description on paper, especially the time or percent effort assigned to each mission, because your requirements for promotion and the level of expectation are directly linked to these assignments, and you need to be accountable. Also, make sure your job description correlates with the reality of what you do on a daily basis so that you can reasonably meet your targets.

Table 2.2 List of potential tracks to promotion

Promotion track	Description/focus
"Triple Threat" clinician-scientist-educator (Tenure accruing)	In addition to excellence in clinical activities, exceptional research (basic science) accomplishments (multiple grants, prolific publication, and mentorship) AND exceptional educational accomplishments (clerkship director, program director, stellar student/resident evaluations, programmatic development, and publication in education field)
Clinician-scientist (Tenure accruing)	In addition to excellence in clinical activities, exceptional research (basic science) accomplishments (multiple extramural grants, program project involvement, prolific presentations and publication (high impact), research mentorship, and service in college/department research mission)
Clinician-scholar	In addition to excellence in clinical activities, substantial (but less than above) academic/research activities (may focus on clinical trial or translational research activities, health services/outcomes research, or intramural quality improvement programs)
Clinician-educator	In addition to excellence in clinical activities, exceptional educational leadership and accomplishments (mentorship, student clerkship director, residency/fellowship program director, stellar student/resident evaluations, programmatic development, service in college/department educational mission, and funding and publication in education field)
Clinician-administrator	In addition to excellence in clinical activities, some substantial administrative duties at the college (i.e., Dean's office, committees) or department (i.e., division/section chief, center director) level
Clinician	Primarily excellence in clinical productivity (recognized expert in field, clinical awards, establishment of a clinical program, RVU goals, mortality/morbidity, quality improvement programs, and other metrics); likely some clinical research
Research	Generally reserved for a non-clinical, strictly research faculty evaluated for excellence in basic science research (multiple extramural grants, laboratory management, prolific presentations and publication (high impact), and mentorship)

The expectations for superior accomplishment in research are both the most challenging and most stringent, but are also the most variable between institutions. The general expectations focus on extramural funding, publication, and mentorship. For some, a career development grant would be enough, while for others, one or more R01 independent investigator grants would be required. For some, 2–3 publications per year would be sufficient, while for others, 4–5 first- or senior- author papers per year specifically in high-impact journals would be required. The *Journal of Surgical Research* (IF = 2.176) is a great place to publish early findings to initially establish yourself and get national exposure. Next, higher-impact surgical journals (Table 2.3) should be your target, with the eventual goal of publishing in the highest-impact clinical and science journals overall (i.e., *New England Journal of Medicine* (34.83), *Cell* (31.15), *Nature* (30.98), *Science* (29.75)). Finally, for some, mentoring T32 residents would be sufficient, while for others, primary mentorship for PhD graduate students would be required. Therefore, know your specific targets and get working early writing grants and publishing – the cliché "publish or perish" may not be literally accurate but for some institutions is not far from reality. Mentorship from a basic scientist outside your division/department is critical to success.

Superior accomplishment in education is focused on mentorship and exceptional teaching commitment primarily to medical students, but also to the surgical residents and fellows. Education has traditionally been less rewarded, but is becoming more recognized, and likely expectations vary less between institutions. Creation of an Education Portfolio, if not required by your institution, is critically important to establish your credentials and accomplishments as a surgical educator. This formal portfolio includes the following components: (1) education philosophy statement; (2) professional development achievements; (3) teaching activity reports; (4) curriculum development accomplishments; (5) teaching effectiveness; (6) advisees and mentees; (7) education administration; and (8) scholarly activity. Appointment as the medical student clerkship director, residency/fellowship program director, or other prominent educational position is important. Teaching awards for consistently

Table 2.3 Top-rated surgical journals by impact factor

Journal	2009 Impact factor
Annals of Surgery	7.90
American Journal of Transplantation	6.43
Endoscopy	5.46
Journal of Neurology, Neurosurgery and Psychiatry	4.87
Archives of Surgery	4.32
Annals of Surgical Oncology	4.13
British Journal of Surgery	4.08
American Journal of Surgical Pathology	4.06
Surgery for Obesity and Related Diseases	3.86
Liver Transplantation	3.72

Adapted from Science Watch (http://sciencewatch.com/dr/sci/10/jul4-10_2/)

achieving above-average to exceptional evaluation scores from students and trainees would be expected. This is an area where service at this early stage at the college level in curriculum committees, advisory groups to the Dean, simulation centers, educational retreats, etc., may be important. In addition, educational curriculum development is important, and this may include local programs or extramurally funded initiatives that may be more regional or national. Involvement in student interest groups, being a student advisor, regular participation in small-group leadership or core lectures, teaching in preclinical courses, etc., all add to your educational portfolio. Unless you are a classically trained educator, you may require mentorship from a professional educator at your institution for success here.

Superior clinical accomplishment involves being recognized as an expert in your field at least locally/regionally, but for some, at least the beginnings of national recognition may be required. Expert technical skills should be backed up by exceptional morbidity and mortality outcomes. You will likely also be required to lead a quality improvement initiative and may need to initiate a novel clinical program in your area of expertise. I think this is the area where most young surgeons are knowledgeable and confident, but mentorship, in this case often from your division chief, is critical to success.

A word about tenure. Tenure and promotion often go hand-in-hand and are affectionately called the "T&P process." Tenure is loosely defined as "the status of holding one's position on a permanent basis without periodic contract renewal." A detailed discussion is beyond the scope of this chapter, but both the true value as well as the relevance of tenure are being called into question in many institutions. Also, many institutions are realigning to offer less tenured positions overall and therefore have made requirements for tenure very rigorous. In Table 2.2, an indication tenure track is included where most likely offered. This is often limited to faculty with exceptional accomplishment in basic science research. Like prior advice, know your specific institution's tenure accruing and non-tenure accruing tracks, and what additional levels of accomplishment may be required to attain both tenure and promotion. The ranges of targets listed above may still be relevant as a starting point. For many surgeons, a clinical non-tenure track may be appropriate and promotion is still achievable independent of tenure, but recognize that tenure or non-tenure designation is usually determined at the time of your initial contract, so be confident you are on the right track.

Independent of the track you are on, mentorship and guidance along the way are keys to success. Make sure your department has a well-defined, structured academic development program for junior faculty. This should be above and beyond the mentorship you get from research and clinical mentors. It should provide you with a basic strategy with goals and milestones that will ensure you will achieve all the necessary targets for promotion. This should include at least annual review of your progress. It should also include a formal mid-career review. Time requirements to promotion vary between institutions and between promotion tracks, but at what constitutes mid-career (3 years in many situations), you should have a comprehensive review including assembling a mock promotion package for formal review within the department and perhaps even the Dean's office in some cases. This is a critical process to review your specific career objectives and promotion targets, to assess progress in all key areas, to identify areas where there may be deficiency that can be addressed over the remaining time, and to re-evaluate as to whether your job description and time allocations match your activities. Take this process and its findings very seriously.

Career Development Awards (CDAs)

The NIH offers a range of awards aimed at providing funding and support for protected time and concentrated research career development (Table 2.4). The VA also offers career development awards (http://www.research.va.gov/funding/cdp.cfm).

The NIH awards generally provide support for 5 years including $50,000–75,000 per year in salary support for the young investigator in exchange for a commitment that 75 % effort be directed to the research supported by the grant. They also provide $25,000–50,000 per year in research funding for supplies and equipment, and travel

Table 2.4 Select NIH career development award options for young investigators

NIH mechanism	Description
K01	Mentored Research Scientist Development Award (Parent K01)
	Provides support and "protected time" (3–5 years) for a young PhD scientist for an intensive, supervised career development experience in the biomedical, behavioral, or clinical sciences leading to research independence
K07	Academic Career Award (Parent K07)
	Provides support for more junior candidates who are interested in developing academic and research expertise
K08	Mentored Clinical Scientist Research Career Development Award (Parent K08)
	Provides support and "protected time" to individuals with a clinical doctoral degree for an intensive, supervised research career development experience in the fields of biomedical and behavioral research, including translational research
K23	Mentored Patient-Oriented Research Career Development Award (Parent K23)
	Provides support for the career development of investigators who have made a commitment to focus their research endeavors on patient-oriented research generally defined as involving patients you treat clinically in clinical or translational research
K99/R00	NIH Pathway to Independence Award (Parent K99/R00)
	Provides an opportunity for promising postdoctoral scientists to receive both mentored and independent research support from the same award. The initial phase will provide 1–2 years of mentored support for highly promising, postdoctoral research scientists followed by up to 3 years of independent support contingent on securing an independent research position

Adapted from National Institutes of Health (http://grants.nih.gov/training/careerdevelopmentawards.htm)

associated with the project. In addition, many professional societies, in collaboration with the American College of Surgeons, offer additional support for K-awardees up to an additional $75,000 per year for salary or expenses, so investigate whether there is one of these matching opportunities relevant for you. CDAs are likely the best, if not only, way for a young surgical investigator to get a foot in the door at NIH. If you already have a PhD and have preliminary data, going direct to an R01 mechanism is preferred. For the others, the ultimate goal for both the investigator and the NIH is to transition preliminary data acquired into a competitive R01 application by the end of the K-award period. If you are contemplating applying for a K-award, planning to do so by the third year of your faculty appointment is generally both advisable and doable. You should have identified a mentor and generated enough preliminary data to that point, and it still gives you enough time to show productivity by the time the promotion process begins.

The K08 and K23 mechanisms are most relevant, with the K08 thought to be for more basic science pursuits, and the K23 for more clinical or translational patient-oriented research. The NIH defines patient-oriented as "research conducted with human subjects (or on material of human origin such as tissues, specimens and cognitive phenomena) for which an investigator directly interacts with human subjects." Whichever mechanism you choose, realize there are pros and cons of these awards. First, make sure your division and department are committed to you spending 75% of your time on research. Make sure you are committed to this as well. Second, since $75,000 may not be 75% of your salary, make sure there are funds outside of clinical activity available to support your time. Third, realize that if you agree to a 75% research assignment, you will need to show research productivity in line with basic science colleagues who may have fewer other responsibilities or distractions. This may set a high bar for promotion on a scientist track. Finally, make sure you know whether or not just having a K-award is enough to qualify you for promotion or whether or not an R01 is mandatory.

The nice part of the CDAs is the career development part itself. You are asked to identify weaknesses in your research portfolio and then design a curriculum to address these weaknesses through courses, training, and the like. This is an opportunity for some to explore and learn new scientific methodology, experience novel techniques, and even travel to learn from experts in the field. This is also another opportunity to consider whether or not the pursuit of an additional degree is desired or necessary. Many institutions have Master's programs in either public health or in clinical and translational research where you can acquire additional skills in epidemiology, biostatistics, or other areas relevant to your program. These degrees are not necessary for a K-award, and the K-award is not necessary for participation in a Master's program, but they are nicely compatible.

Another nice avenue through which to pursue academic career development is through involvement in academic and professional societies like the Association for Academic Surgery (AAS). The benefit is multi-faceted. First, you will meet new colleagues who have the same career goals as you and who will face the same promotion process. These people will become friends, advisors, mentors, and potential research collaborators along the way. Second, you get to present your research, often preliminary, in a constructive setting where you get critical feedback and an opportunity to cross-pollinate ideas to improve or expand your activities. Third, these societies offer courses, like the Fundamentals of Surgical Research Course or Career Development Course offered by the AAS, which provide you with the basic foundation on which to build your early academic career. And finally, they provide the opportunity for you to get involved in society organization and governance which allows you to start building a national reputation even early in your career.

Contemplating a Mid-Career Move?

At or about that 3-year mid-career mark, you may be contemplating a move to a different faculty position. The reasons for this vary. Some may be dissatisfied with their current position, realizing the process outlined above didn't produce a good fit, and have concerns about achieving their goals in that environment. Others may have had a good fit, but things (i.e., leadership, department mission or focus, mentors, etc.) may have changed negatively impacting the environment. Still others may use a move as a mechanism to garner early promotion, thinking that they may have achieved milestones ahead of schedule. If you truly deserve a vertical move to associate professor, then it may be OK to pursue it, but avoid using this latter approach just to advance your title. In any case, moving at this stage can be very disruptive – you are just establishing roots in your first position, and pulling them up will set you back at least a year. It may be the right move and the "grass may indeed be greener" in the new position, but just realize it is a significant decision, so get advice from those that know you best.

Approaching Promotion

Hopefully there is an organized process as part of the department academic development program to help walk you through the promotion paperwork process because it can be very demanding and confusing. One thing you can do to help yourself from the beginning is to establish a folder (either physical file folder or virtual computer folder) in which to place all information relevant to your promotion packet. You can place abstracts, manuscripts, invitations to speak at conferences, evaluations, etc., in this folder real-time so it doesn't get lost and can be relatively easily organized for your application when the time comes. At the mid-career review, you can begin to organize this material, but keep collecting everything that may have bearing on your packet right up until it is submitted. A full discussion of the actual promotion application process is beyond the scope of this chapter and varies so much from institution to institution that I refer you to the information provided by your own institution locally.

A few important highlights are worth mentioning. In addition to having the foresight to be organized and collect information real-time, another semi-conscious way to do the same is to compulsively keep your curriculum vitae (CV) up to date. Much of the information from your CV can then be cut and pasted into the promotion packet template. Start organizing your packet early and get help because these templates are not always intuitive, and it is at times hard to figure out which information goes where. Know all the important deadlines along the application process so that you don't miss a critical submission. In general, the packet is composed of sections for each of the areas of expertise – patient care, teaching, research, and service. In addition to a list of your accomplishments, you will need to provide personal statements detailing your clinical, research, and educational philosophies. Be enthusiastic, organized, clear, and concise. Next, make sure you have accurate documentation of any and all funding, peer-review activities, manuscripts, abstracts submitted, presentations given (both peer-reviewed and invited), students or residents mentored, data regarding your evaluations, and any academic honors you have received. This process should be an accurate accounting of all of the hard work you have put in over the last 6 or more years. The final component is to solicit letters of recommendation from people of prominence around the country who know you well and whose support will register soundly with the promotion committee. Again requirements vary, but you will generally need a balanced list of approximately five internal recommendations and five external recommendations. These should ideally be people who have achieved full professor at their own institutions and who have attained significant academic and national stature, but also people who know you well enough to lend strong personal support to your application. Again, start this process early because such people are often busy and need time to complete your letter, and don't be afraid to send reminders as the deadline approaches to be sure your application is complete.

Associate Professor and Transition to Full Professor

Now that you have achieved promotion to Associate Professor, do not let up on your effort. Your accomplishments as Assistant Professor serve as the springboard that will propel you to Full Professor and the process starts right away. The timeline to Professor is usually less well defined than for your first promotion. In general, if you have stayed right on track, you should be eligible for Professor at about the 10-year mark into your academic career or roughly 4–5 years after your promotion to Associate. The main focus of this next stage should be the establishment of your expertise and reputation *nationally* (and even internationally). Clinically, this may involve the establishment of a unique clinical program in your field that effects practice patterns, active clinical trial activity and leadership, and/or important high-impact clinical publications in the field. This may lead to an invitation to participate in American Board of Surgery activities. National recognition in research will come primarily through establishing yourself as an independent investigator with multiple extramural grants. You will need to keep up momentum in this regard and write and submit grants and publish regularly. Your national recognition and expertise in research will be rewarded by invitations to serve on NIH study sections. Further national recognition in academics will come through increased involvement in professional societies like the AAS or Society for University Surgeons and demonstration of significant leadership positions including holding officer positions. National recognition on education can be achieved through the establishment of novel educational curricula that get national exposure and perhaps adoption through societies like the Association for Surgical Education, the Accreditation Council for Graduate Medical Education, and the American College of Surgeons. Educationally, this is also a time to increase mentorship activities both locally and nationally and truly impact the next generation of surgeons. Finally, this is the time where you may consider some of the opportunities that you passed on previously like service locally on committees (i.e., the Institutional Review Board, the Institutional Animal Care and Use Committee, medical school curriculum committees, or clinical QI or operating room committees), heavier participation in textbook chapter or editorial contributions, and editorial activity on specialty journals. Hopefully, with this continued effort and success will come a regular stream of invitations to speak nationally and even internationally to effectively solidify your reputation as expert in the field.

Conclusion

There is no one prescription for guaranteed success in academic surgery, but clearly knowing and understanding the requirements for promotion, setting yourself up initially with the necessary resources and mentorship to get started, proactively protecting and organizing your time, and then demonstrating a tenacious work ethic in pursuit of grant funding and manuscript publication will serve you well. Define early what your primary mission in addition to clinical productivity will be – basic science research, clinical research, or education – and then work hard to establish expertise in that area that will satisfy promotion. Several other chapters in this book cover topics (i.e., mentorship, grant and manuscript writing, setting up a research program/research team, time management, and work-life balance) that are intimately linked and synergistic to the material provided here to provide a comprehensive framework for success.

Acknowledgments I would like to acknowledge lectures given at the AAS Fall Courses over the years on topics covered in this chapter by the following surgeons: Drs. Charles Balch, Anees Chagpar, Herbert Chen, N. Joseph Espat, Clark Gamblin, Steven Hughes, James McGinty, George Sarosi, C. Max Schmidt, Sharon Weber, and Stephen Yang.

Selected Reading

1. Baumgartner WA, Tseng EE, DeAngelis CD. Training women surgeons and their academic advancement. Ann Thorac Surg. 2001;71(2 Suppl):S22–4.
2. Klingensmith ME, Anderson KD. Educational scholarship as a route to academic promotion: a depiction of surgical education scholars. Am J Surg. 2006;191:533–7.
3. Sanfey H. Promotion to professor: a career development resource. Am J Surg. 2010;200:554–7.
4. Souba WW, Gamelli RL, Lorber MI, et al. Strategies for success in academic surgery. Surgery. 1995;117:90–5.
5. Thompson RW, Schucker B, Kent KC, et al. Reviving the vascular surgeon-scientist: an interim assessment of the jointly sponsored Lifeline Foundation/National Heart, Lung, and Blood Institute William J. von Liebig Mentored Clinical Scientist Development (K08) Program. J Vasc Surg. 2007;45(Suppl):A2–7.

Part II
Research: From Conception to Publication

Chapter 3
Reviewing the Literature, Developing a Hypothesis, Study Design

Rosalie Carr and C. Max Schmidt

Introduction

Initiation of any research investigation requires proper preparation and planning. A thorough review of the literature is essential on your topic of interest. With this accomplished, one may reasonably develop original and relevant (i.e., meaningful) hypotheses. Not all original and relevant hypotheses, however, are feasible (i.e., testable). Once a relevant, and feasible hypothesis has been developed, an optimal study may be designed to prove or disprove the hypothesis. A study may use quantitative, or mixed. An optimal study should be adequately powered, free of bias, and be able to be conducted in a reasonable timeframe with resources available to the investigator.

Reviewing the Literature

A thorough review of the literature on your topic of interest is essential. Prior to reviewing the literature, however, one must pick a topic of interest. Choice of your topic of interest may directly facilitate a thorough review of the literature. The topic of interest should optimally be as ***narrow*** as possible. This will facilitate a thorough review of the literature on the topic and subsequent mastery of the subject matter. A broad topic, conversely, will be cumbersome to review and may not result in true mastery of the subject matter.

A proper review of the literature uses ***multiple sources*** of information on the topic of interest. These resources include original peer-reviewed papers, textbooks,

---

R. Carr, M.D. • C.M. Schmidt, M.D., Ph.D., M.B.A., F.A.C.S. (✉)
Department of Surgery, Biochemistry and Molecular Biology, Indiana University School of Medicine, 980 W Walnut St C522, Indianapolis, IN 46202, USA

chapters, reviews, editorials, but also online and personal resources, e.g., experts in the field. Most important of these, however, are original, peer-reviewed papers. Textbooks, chapters, reviews, editorials, and online resources, while helpful in identifying primary sources of information on your topic and organizing large amounts of information, should not be weighed heavily in your literature review. These resources notoriously contain significant bias on the subject matter.

In order to perform a thorough review of original peer-reviewed papers, a *Medline* search of all relevant works is an excellent first step. Investigators should have a low threshold to use the library staff at their institution/university to insure proper Subject and Medical Subject Headings (MeSH) terms and headings are used. The quality of the original work should be reviewed in a systematic fashion. Questions to address when reviewing an original work in the literature (or designing a study) are:

1. *Internally valid?*
2. *Externally valid?*
3. *Appropriate conclusions?*

An *internally valid* study is adequately powered and free from selection, time, and information bias. It is also free of misclassification errors and confounding variables. *Adequate power* is particularly important when no significant effect is demonstrated in a study under review. For negative studies, it is critical to appreciate whether there was an adequate sample size to determine a significant difference in the parameter being assessed. Otherwise, "no effect" is an invalid conclusion. Such an error is called a Beta error, or Type II error. This is related to power by the formula, Power = 1-Beta, where Beta is the chance that one fails to detect a difference when one exists. *Selection bias* is when subjects in treatment groups are not selected randomly, e.g., the investigator chooses which patients to enroll on study. *Time bias* is when subjects in one treatment have the advantage or disadvantage of time. An example of *lead time bias* is when patients who have colon cancers detected on screening colonoscopy live longer than patients who actually developed symptoms prior to colon cancer detection. Colonoscopy does not result in longer life from colon cancer; rather, when screening examinations reveal cancer, they simply detect the cancer sooner. *Information bias* is when the data collection is not equivalent between groups (e.g., derived from individuals, or with). *Misclassification errors* are when treatments or groups are incorrectly assigned due to suboptimal classification, e.g., if the study relies on subjective recall of past events. Finally, *confounding variables* may invalidate a study. Confounding variables are variables in the treatment groups that result in the 'effect' or the "non-effect" being studied. For example, patients undergoing abdominal CT scan compared to patients who have not undergone CT scan have a higher incidence of gastrointestinal. CT does not cause the gastrointestinal disorder, but rather is associated with gastrointestinal disorders because it is commonly employed to diagnose them.

Assessment of internal validity can only be performed if sufficient information about the study design is given within the report. If the study design description does not allow a thorough evaluation of the study's freedom from bias, then it cannot be determined internally valid. Therefore quality of reporting is a factor in study validity.

An *externally valid* study is one where the results actually have *meaning* beyond the numbers and may be *generalizable* to other like populations. The external validity largely depends upon the inclusion and exclusion criteria, but also depends upon the study population. If the study population is unique, it may not be broadly applicable to other populations even if they meet the inclusion and exclusion criteria. Clinical relevance may also affect the external validity of a study. Even though the results may be statistically significant, the effect may be so small that it is not actually *meaningful* in the real world. Finally, sometimes the results may be statistically significant, but not actually real. Finding a difference when no difference exists is termed an *alpha error, or a Type I error*, e.g., p-value (alpha) = 0.05. This indicates a 5 % chance that the difference detected between two or more groups is due to random chance rather than a true effect.

Finally, after reviewing the internal validity and external validity of a study, one must make sure that the authors of the study have drawn *appropriate conclusions*. Randomized controlled trials may actually determine cause and effect relationships whereas other studies may only determine association.

Another type of bias to consider when performing a complete review of the literature is *publication bias*. This bias results when study publication is dependent upon the results. Recent literature reports that studies with positive or statistically significant results are more likely to be published. If negative results are published, they tend to take longer to be accepted for publication which leads to *time lag bias*. Because those studies are initially missing from the literature, incorrect conclusions are made. Ideally, all research should be published, or should at least be represented within published data. Even with a complete review of the literature, publication bias makes it difficult to arrive at an accurate understanding of a topic due to underrepresentation of negative studies.

Once you have researched the topic with all available resources, *consulting with experts in the field* is essential as it may help overcome misconceptions based on publication bias. Individuals who have studied or practiced in the field of interest will have assimilated the relevant information on multiple occasions and may have a perspective one cannot glean from reviewing the literature on one occasion in isolation.

With a proper and thorough review of the literature, one will become an expert in the subject matter. With this expertise, an original and relevant hypothesis is most likely to be developed.

Developing a Hypothesis

With a thorough review of the literature accomplished, one may reasonably develop original and relevant (i.e., meaningful) hypotheses. The hypothesis should be original so there is not unnecessary duplication of research. Repeating a study may indeed have merit, e.g., if the control population was suboptimal in the original study or if there was inadequate power and the original study failed to demonstrate a difference in the parameters under study. Simply repeating a study for the sake of repeating it, however, is not optimal in terms of resource utilization and really needs to be justified based on concerns of improving the original design. In addition to original, the hypothesis should be relevant. A relevant hypothesis is one that once proven true or false should result in a change in behavior for the betterment of mankind. Consider the following hypothesis: individuals who are left-handed are able to perform right-handed tasks better than right-handed individuals perform left-handed tasks. It is unclear how such a hypothesis is relevant and will result in any change in behavior for the betterment of mankind. A hypothesis may be relevant, but not feasible (i.e., able to be tested). A hypothesis may not be testable due to statistical or ethical considerations. Consider the following hypothesis: individuals with a rare condition (that affects only two individuals in the world) have significant symptom resolution with treatment A vs. B vs. C. Such a study is not feasible since there are only two individuals (N=2) that may be tested. Consider another hypothesis: routine catheterization of the carotid artery in humans results in more accurate blood pressure determination than radial artery catheterization. This study is not testable due to being prohibited on ethical grounds.

With these caveats in mind, the steps to *creating a hypothesis* are as follows:

1. **Define the question.**
2. **Define the population.**
3. **Define the intervention.**
4. **Define the results.**
5. **Define the next question.**

In developing a hypothesis, a *principal or primary question* needs to be identified. Once identified, the principal or primary question needs to be defined precisely. A precise definition will involve:

1. *Description of intervention(s) and treatment group(s), e.g., resection vs. observation*
2. *Response variables, e.g., quality of life, survival, disease-free survival*
3. *Measurement methods for response variables and group comparisons*

Secondary questions should optimally be defined from the outset as well. There should be a limited number of secondary questions, to avoid significantly increasing the risk of an alpha error, i.e., finding a difference when no difference exists. In any analysis of data, statistical corrections should be performed to account for multiple comparisons, e.g., Bonferroni adjustment.

After defining the principal question, the population needs to be defined. The *reference population* may be all patients with a given condition, e.g., pancreatic adenocarcinoma. The *available population* may be all patients with pancreatic adenocarcinoma at Indiana University. The *eligible population* may be all patients with pancreatic adenocarcinoma at Indiana University who are aware of and eligible for the study. Finally, the *study population* are those eligible patients who actually enroll on study. The study population must be representative of the reference population in order for the study to be internally valid. If the final study participant population varies significantly from the reference population, then conclusions about that reference population cannot be made based on the results of the study.

After defining the study population, the *specific intervention* (what, who, when and how) and *anticipated or expected results* need to be defined. Writing the anticipated/expected results section prior to initiating any study will help to guide experiments and facilitate the study design. The most appropriate outcome variables and the best method to measure these outcome variables will in this manner be defined.

Given the anticipated results of the study, defining the *next question* or the follow-up question to the principal question is important. This gives the study purpose within a greater framework, i.e., determines its broader applicability. Defining the next question is also important for written or oral presentation of the study and justification of a grant for funding of the study.

The hypothesis must then be phrased so that it may be either proved or disproved; it must be "falsifiable." Every hypothesis has a "null hypothesis" which is the condition in which the hypothesis is disproved, or the default position in which no difference exists between the variables being studied. A well-crafted hypothesis will lead to a study design that will either prove or disprove the hypothesis.

Study Design

Once a feasible and relevant hypothesis has been developed, an optimal study may be designed to prove or disprove your hypothesis.

Questions to address when designing a study are identical to those addressed above in the section on reviewing the literature. An optimal study should be constructed so it is internally and externally valid. The study should be adequately powered, free of bias, and able to be conducted in a reasonable timeframe with resources available to the investigator.

In order to determine if your study has adequate power, a *power analysis* needs to be performed. *Power* is the probability of finding a significant difference when a difference does indeed exist. A power calculation is complicated and likely should be performed in consultation with a biostatistician. Nonetheless, there are free software programs available online to familiarize one with the technique.

http://biostat.mc.vanderbilt.edu/PowerSampleSize

The essential aspects of any power analysis include:

1. *Type of test (e.g., T-test)*
2. *Alpha error (e.g., 0.05)*
3. *Sample size*
4. *Estimated effect size*

A power calculation estimates sample size needed to yield valuable results. If the study is underpowered with too small a sample size, results are likely to be meaningless. Conversely, a sample size greater than necessary can be wasteful and put subjects at unnecessary risk.

Effect size is a way to standardize measurement of a treatment effect, so it may be compared to other treatments targeted at the same outcome. Effect size also allows one to estimate whether statistically significant effects are actually relevant or ***meaningful***. If the outcome of interest is a categorical variable, effect size is the difference in the proportion of patients with that outcome between treatment and control groups. If the outcome of interest is a continuous variable, effect size is the difference in means (of that outcome) between treatment and control divided by the standard deviation of the control. The following is a rough guide to interpretation of the effect size:

<0.3 = small effect
0.3–0.5 = moderate effect
>0.5 = large difference effect

The effect size is unknown in the design of a trial, so one must estimate the effect size. By convention, a value of 0.5 (moderate effect) is used in power calculations. When all values are entered into the power formula, a value (0–1) will result. In general, if the result is <0.8, sample size is inadequate to fully power the study.

Bias can never be fully excluded in any study, but it must be minimized as much as possible. Community paradigms and the researchers own personality and biography often impede objectivity. Researchers hold pre-existing beliefs which may cause them to see in their results confirmation of these beliefs. ***Confirmation bias***, looking for a preconceived result despite contrary findings should be avoided. Responsible conduct of research, or ***research integrity***, has been a popular topic in recent literature. One major component is presenting all relevant data and analyses instead of arranging/omitting data to support the most favorable hypothesis. Selection of results chosen for publication based on the nature of results, most often results that are statistically significant, is called ***outcome reporting bias.***

Time to complete a study, if prolonged, may result in the introduction of significant time bias as new technologies and approaches will inevitably develop. Finally, if personnel, and resources are not available to the investigator, then the trial will likely fail to achieve its objectives.

Any research investigation initiative should start by asking the question: Is a randomized controlled trial possible? Randomized controlled trials are difficult to perform logistically in rare diseases. They are also difficult to perform where strong community bias (ethical or otherwise) exists for a particular treatment or existing data is compelling for one treatment over another. ***Randomized controlled trials*** provide the highest level of data followed by prospective cohort, retrospective case control studies, and other trials. Randomized controlled trials may actually determine cause and effect relationships whereas other studies may only determine association. Any study less rigorous than a randomized controlled trial has significant potential for bias and confounders.

In addition to all of the above, to design an optimal study, ***consulting with experts in the field*** is essential. Individuals who have studied or practiced in the field of interest will have assimilated the relevant information on multiple occasions and may have a perspective one cannot glean from reviewing the literature on one occasion in isolation. Make sure that you have adequate resources and mentorship before venturing into any study.

Research is about discovering the truth. Revel in the mystery and joy of discovery whether or not your hypothesis is correct. If done carefully, your contribution to mankind may be immeasurable.

Acknowledgements Carl Schmidt, MD, MSCI
  Assistant Professor Surgery
  The Ohio State University

Financial Support Indiana Genomics Initiative (INGEN) of Indiana University. INGEN is supported in part by Lilly Endowment Inc. (CMS)

Suggested Additional Reading

1. Friedman LM, et al. Fundamentals of clinical trials. 4th ed. 2010.
2. Hulley SB. Designing clinical research. 4th ed. 2013.
3. Penson, Wei. Clinical research methods for surgeons. 2006.
4. Piantadosi S. Clinical trials: a methodological perspective. 2nd ed. 2005.

Chapter 4
Ethics in Surgical Research

Richard A. Burkhart and Timothy M. Pawlik

Introduction

The ethical practice of both medicine and research remains a cornerstone of the physician's duty. The physician-patient relationship is dependent upon sound ethics and good judgment. This is especially true when patients invest in clinical or translational research efforts to further medical knowledge. Ethical decision-making is particularly relevant in surgical research, where goals are extended beyond the development of novel drug therapies to include the evaluation of new technologies and techniques. Further, as surgeons take the lead in quality improvement initiatives, the ethical principles of the research environment must be taken into account as health systems and processes are changed. As a surgeon, these additional research aims require a nuanced understanding of ethical principles beyond those required of our non-surgical colleagues. Ethical concerns around clinical research include informed consent, respect for autonomy, an acceptable risk-benefit ratio, and ensuring that the research is scientifically rigorous enough to justify human subject involvement. Investigators involved in basic science research frequently find themselves confronted with issues of honesty and objectivity, multiple conflicts of interest, as well as controversy regarding authorship and publication of data. Investigators involved in quality improvement initiatives often strive to understand the risk conveyed to patients, identify and define rigorous outcome measures for study, and determine the level of ethical oversight and review board involvement required for the work. Learning to identify and handle ethical issues in research is an important skill for academic surgeons. Ethical conduct of

R.A. Burkhart, M.D.
Department of Surgery, Johns Hopkins University School of Medicine,
Baltimore, MD, USA

T.M. Pawlik, M.D., M.P.H., Ph.D. (✉)
Department of Surgery, The Ohio State University Wexner Medical Center,
Columbus, OH, USA

surgical research is not only part of each surgeon's professional identify, but also defines us as leaders among peers. Although an exhaustive review of the ethical issues involved in surgical research is beyond the scope of this chapter, we herein highlight the main ethical issues that arise in the setting of surgical research.

The Dual Loyalties of the Surgeon-Scientist

Research is an important aspect of the surgeon-scientist identity. As clinicians we have a duty to place the needs of our patients above all else. As investigators, we have a duty to future patients who may benefit from our research. The goals of research can sometimes conflict with our fiduciary duty to the individual patient in front of us. Furthermore, personal gain from research discoveries (even just the extreme satisfaction of benefiting a large number of future patients or advancing science, not-withstanding academic advancement) can bias our personal assessment about what is right.

In effect, the surgeon-scientist can find him/herself in the role of double-agent: surgeon versus scientist. This problem is exemplified by the story of William Beaumont [1]. A young military surgeon, Dr. Beaumont acutely treated and saved the life of the French-Canadian fur trapper, Alexis St. Martin in 1822. St. Martin was injured when his shotgun accidentally discharged at close range leaving him with a gaping hole in his abdomen. Due in large part to Dr. Beaumont's surgical care, St. Martin survived the incident, but was left with a persistent gastro-cutaneous fistula. Over the next 20 years, Beaumont and St. Martin shared a unique relationship dominated by Beaumont's dual loyalties. While Beaumont continued to care for his "patient," he also performed multiple studies to define the physiology of the stomach using St. Martin as his research subject. In turn, Beaumont advanced critical knowledge about the functioning of the stomach and benefitted professionally from this relationship as he went on to help define the theory of how humans digest their meals in his landmark publication, *"Experiments and Observations of the Gastric Juice and the Physiology of Digestion"*. Unfortunately, the relationship between Beaumont and St. Martin evolved as St. Martin became healthy enough to not need Beaumont's constant supervision and care. At multiple points during their patient-doctor relationship St. Martin dissolved their relationship in order to put an end to Beaumont's uncomfortable and frequently painful experiments. Nonetheless, Beaumont used his special position as St. Martin's doctor to coerce his patient to participate in additional studies.

The example of Dr. Beaumont and Mr. St. Martin highlights the conflicted loyalties of the surgeon-scientist. Not infrequently our goal to advance surgical science can compete with our responsibility for patient care. This conflict is inherent in the enterprise of surgical research and is particularly prominent in clinical trials and other human subjects research. Specifically, as we act in our traditional fiduciary role as care-providers, we must also be cognizant of how the goals of research and scientific discovery can impact our actions and decisions. While the conflict of dual loyalties cannot be completely eliminated, it can be managed through safeguards to protect the interests of patients. For example, principal investigators should avoid personally consenting and enrolling their own patients in their clinical trials. In addition, surgeon-scientists should constantly re-evaluate who the stakeholders are in the research environment and who serves to benefit from the interaction or intervention.

Management of the problem of dual-loyalties will be case specific and needs to be individualized based on the context of the clinical and research circumstance. It is important to recognize that even the perception that the surgeon scientist is not acting in the best interest of his or her patient can erode the foundation of trust in the physician-patient relationship. As such, it is critical that surgeon-scientists are aware of the potential problem of dual-loyalties so that it can be recognized and managed. Additional management strategies for the problem of dual-loyalties include transparency, full-disclosure, and possible third-party mediation/facilitation.

At times, a surgeon may in fact be asked to serve as the third-party mediator, or facilitator, for other research endeavors. In these cases, dual loyalties can extend beyond the surgeon's own research and include situations where the surgeon acts as a gatekeeper for patient recruitment in others' research endeavors. This is an increasingly frequent scenario as multi-institutional and multi-investigator alliances are formed to investigate relatively rare diseases or increasingly specific subsets of more common disease presentations. Particularly when surgical care represents the gold-standard for current therapy (as is frequently the case in early-stage oncologic disease, operative trauma, and many other areas of general surgery), the recruitment of patients into clinical trials will often take place in a surgical setting. In this role, surgeons (along with potential bias and conflicts of interest) have the capacity to either inhibit or increase trial enrollment. There are instances where a surgeon may be incentivized to participate (either through the potential for academic advancement or even at times through financial gain). In other cases, surgeons may be apt to not participate due to a lack of incentive (perhaps allowing a patient and third party investigator to occupy a clinic room for an additional hour may be detrimental to other patients or the health system in general). A participating surgeon-scientist must recognize the ethical questions and potential for bias raised by physician incentives when acting as a gatekeeper in research. Finally, as a gatekeeper, it is imperative that the surgeon-scientist be well versed in the risk-benefit profile of the proposed research and ensures that research is conducted with the health and safety of the patient foremost in mind.

In addition to the problem of dual loyalties, professional judgment regarding the best interest of the patient can be unduly influenced by secondary concerns such as career advancement or even financial gain. In an environment often defined by "publish or perish" the surgeon-scientist is required to be academically productive. Although the surgeon-scientist's primary goal is to improve the status of the surgical patient, the academic environment creates a tension whereby surgeon-scientists are driven to produce data, publish, and get promoted.

Human Subject Research

Many academic surgeons are involved in research that directly involves the use of human subjects. Such research may include clinical trials or investigations that introduce new procedures or technologies into the clinical setting. Unfortunately, there are many examples of human subject research that have been characterized by unethical behavior [2]. Many surgeons are familiar with atrocities committed during World War II when the Nazi regime subjected individuals to horrible unethical experiments. The subsequent

Nuremberg trials and Nuremberg code established informed consent as a central tenet to protect human subjects involved in research [3]. The Nuremberg code states that the "voluntary consent of the human subject is absolutely essential." In addition, the Nuremberg code notes that "the experiment should be such as to yield fruitful results for the good of society, unprocurable by other methods or means of study, and not random and unnecessary in nature." [3] In 1964, the World Medical Association adopted the Declaration of Helsinki on the Ethical Principles for Medical Research Involving Human Subjects [4]. The Declaration of Helsinki, which has been subsequently amended, further clarifies the ethical principles for medical research involving human subjects. The Declaration of Helsinki clearly establishes the primacy of individual patient interests over any greater societal good that might be achieve through research. Specifically, the Declaration notes that "the health of the patient will be the first consideration" and that "the well-being of the individual research subject must take precedence over all other interests" [4]. Despite these codes and declarations, multiple examples of unethical research behavior can be identified in the history of the United States. Examples include the well-known unethical Tuskegee Syphilis studies [5] as well as the example at the Jewish Chronic Disease Hospital where 22 elderly patients were injected with live cancer cells by Chester Southam from the Memorial Sloan-Kettering Hospital [6].

Currently, in the United States, the protection of human subjects who participate in research is governed by the United States Department of Health and Human Services Title 45 CFR 46 known as the "The Common Rule" [7]. The Common Rule has four parts which describe basic principles governing human subject research in the general population and among vulnerable populations. Any systematic data collection using human subjects, whether during research development, testing, or evaluation, designed to develop or contribute to generalizable knowledge is considered "human subjects research" and is subject to the Common Rule. In turn, all research using human subjects is required by law to undergo an objective external review to ensure that the research is ethically appropriate, scientifically sound and does not pose undue risk to the participants. This independent review usually takes the form of an institutional review board (IRB). IRBs are comprised of individuals who ensure adequate review of research activities and are typically made up of individuals both from within an institution and from the community. IRBs are charged to (a) evaluate research protocols and determine appropriateness (most commonly providing findings for approval, disapproval, or approval with modification), (b) monitor the progress and conduct of a study, and (c) suspend, terminate, restrict, or request modification to a study as necessary [8]. Investigators have an ethical responsibility not to proceed with human subject research prior to IRB approval. In addition, researchers must report to the IRB any adverse or unanticipated events that may occur over the course of the research. Finally, researchers must participate in annual IRB review and renewal.

In addition to the independent IRB review described above, human subject research must meet other certain minimal requirements in order to be ethical [9, 10]. Emanuel and colleagues have proposed seven key ethical requirements for clinical research (Table 4.1). Research involving human subjects must provide an aggregate benefit to society or future patients to warrant the risk (however small) to current research subjects. In addition, all research should be scientifically valid with robust

Table 4.1 Seven requirements for determining whether a research trial is ethical

Requirement	Explanation	Justifying Ethical Values	Expertise for Evaluation
Social or scientific value	Evaluation of a treatment, intervention, or theory that will improve health and well-being or increase knowledge	Scarce resources and nonexploitation	Scientific knowledge; citizen's understanding of social priorities
Scientific validity	Use of accepted scientific principles and methods, including statistical techniques, to produce reliable and valid data	Scarce resources and nonexploitation	Scientific and statistical knowledge; knowledge of condition and population to assess feasibility
Fair subject selection	Selection of subjects so that stigmatized and vulnerable individuals are not targeted for risky research and the rich and socially powerful not favored for potentially beneficial research	Justice	Scientific knowledge; ethical and legal knowledge
Favorable risk-benefit ratio	Minimization of risks; enhancement of potential benefits; risks to the subject are proportionate to the benefits to the subject and society	Nonmaleficence, beneficence, and nonexploitation	Scientific knowledge; citizen's understanding of social values
Independent review	Review of the design of the research trial, its proposed subject population, and risk-benefit ratio by individuals unaffiliated with the research	Public accountability; minimizing influence of potential conflicts of interest	Intellectual, financial, and otherwise independent researchers; scientific and ethical knowledge
Informed consent	Provision of information to subjects about purpose of the research, its procedures, potential risks, benefits, and alternatives, so that the individual understands this information and can make a voluntary decision whether to enroll and continue to participate	Respect for subject autonomy	Scientific knowledge; ethical and legal knowledge

(continued)

Table 4.1 (continued)

Requirement	Explanation	Justifying Ethical Values	Expertise for Evaluation
Respect for potential and enrolled subjects	Respect for subjects by 1. Permitting withdrawal from the research; 2. Protecting privacy through confidentiality; 3. Informing subjects of newly discovered risks or benefits; 4. Informing subjects of results of clinical research; 5. Maintaining welfare of subjects	Respect for subject autonomy and welfare	Scientific knowledge; ethical and legal knowledge; knowledge of particular subject population

Used with permission, Emanuel et al. [10]
aEthical requirements are listed in chronological order from conception of research to its formulation and implementation

methodology. Researchers must also ensure that all enrolled subjects are shown the highest respect, which is facilitated by the researcher being honest, careful, and transparent with relevant information. Finally, as noted, all human subjects must provide informed consent and be notified that withdrawal from the research study is not only permitted, but will also not affect any aspect of their future care.

Informed Consent

The process of informed consent remains a cornerstone of human subjects research. While not sufficient in itself, informed consent is a necessary prerequisite for virtually all research that involves human subjects. Paramount to the practice of surgery and the conduct of research is the ability to instill trust and facilitate communication. Over the past 50 years, patient autonomy as well as the right to individual self-determination has come to the forefront of medicine and medical research. Informed consent epitomizes the shift toward a patient-centered paradigm of care and clinical research and represents a formal mechanism both to recognize patient autonomy and to address human subjects as self-determined moral agents. Informed consent serves to identify and respect an individual's best interests by giving each person the opportunity to decide autonomously what his or her best interests are in light of the research protocol.

Informed consent is particularly important in the realm of the surgeon-scientist. Research subjects need a significant amount of information to decide whether to enroll in a clinical trial, as many of the attendant risks and benefits are not inherently obvious. At times, researchers must approach patients who are facing significant illness and a bleak prognosis to ask them to participate in a clinical trial. Patients may have a wide range of emotions, from "profound distrust to unquestioned faith" in the surgeon and the research process, thereby further complicating the process [11]. For pragmatic purposes there are three general steps to informed consent: disclosure/information exchange, ensuring adequate understanding/answering of questions, and subject decision-making/consent. Disclosure should convey the relevant and germane information about the study including informing subjects about the purpose of the research, the procedures or medications involved in research, their potential risks, benefits and alternatives [10]. The scope and nature of the information should be determined, in part, by an understanding of the subject's situation and context. This naturally dictates that though an informed consent document may be standardized for each study, the language of the consent process is unique for each potential subject. It is critical that researchers bear in mind that disclosure of information may sometimes be mundane for research personnel, but the process is often novel and confusing for potential participants. As such, information should be presented as clearly as possible with honest admissions of variables that are not well-known or understood. Informed consent may require the use of lay terminology, diagrams, or similar strategies to educate the potential study participant and evaluate that individual's understanding. The language used by the surgeon-scientist in the information disclosure process should be as objective as possible. Surgeons with direct involvement in a clinical trial (either as primary investigator or as potential financial beneficiary) should involve other members of the research team to secure the informed consent process to avoid a potential conflict of interest. Many patients will want their surgeon's subjective opinion of whether they should participate in a specific clinical trial. In general, it is best that the surgeon withhold an opinion until after the research team has met with the potential study participant and discussed the details of the study. By separating the surgeon from the informed consent process for research, the clinical relationship and the surgeons' fiduciary responsibility to the individual patient can be maintained.

Patients can come through the informed consent process without truly being "informed". Having an individual simply sign a consent form to satisfy a legal requirement does not necessarily reflect that the person understands the risks and benefits of a research study. As such, while written consent is a routine and necessary part of the informed consent process, researchers should not overly focus on the paper while ignoring the process. Notwithstanding these comments, the study subject's signature is almost always necessary to proceed with participation in clinical research, and therefore some form of documentation must exist. The informed consent process is critical in respecting human subject autonomy and the right to self-determination as a moral agent. As such, the researcher must ensure that adequate time and priority are allocated for this process.

Surgical Innovation and Surgical Research

Surgeons are uniquely positioned to be innovators in medical therapy, specifically in surgical technique. As most surgeons are constantly tinkering to perfect their intraoperative skills and postoperative outcomes, there is a natural tendency and desire to improve surgical care incrementally. However, the boundaries between tinkering, innovation and research are not always clear cut. A great majority of surgical advancement is the result of surgical innovation, an unregulated process that can spread valuable and effective therapies rapidly but also has the potential to harm patients who are unaware of the innovation in progress. Furthermore, there are a large number of surgical innovations that ultimately proved to be hazardous to patients (historical examples include frontal lobotomy and internal mammary ligation for angina).

It is helpful to define the distinction between innovation and research in order to determine the level of oversight required, as well as patient consent for participation. First, a minor modification (i.e. tinkering) is generally unplanned and involves a slight shift in technique. The evolution of the ileo-anal pull-through with numerous pouch conformations is a good example of a minor modification. It is helpful to remember that surgical research is defined as the systematic investigation of a surgical problem that leads to generalized knowledge. A randomized trial of carotid endarterectomy versus carotid stenting is a good example of surgical research. Innovation is much more difficult to define. The Society of University Surgeons defined innovation as any surgical procedure that has not been described in a North American Surgical text. In addition to endorsing this definition of innovation, the Society of University Surgeons went on to recommend that all innovative procedures must be disclosed ahead of time when planned or discussed postoperatively with patients if the innovation was unplanned [12]. Awareness of the distinction between innovation and minor surgical modification is important for the protection of our patients as, "surgeons must remain alert to the possibility of acceptable clinical innovation, creeping inexorably toward reckless experimentation." [13].

The application of robotic instrumentation in the operating room is a particularly good example of how an evolving modern innovation can be advanced in the context of historical ethical standards [14]. There are several unique aspects of robotic technology that require special attention. The first is the technical capacity to perform a safe operation on a new platform. Similar to the issues navigated during the advent of laparoscopy, complete disclosure and an appropriate risk-benefit analysis must be conveyed during the informed consent process in the context of a surgeon progressing along the learning curve with a new technology. The successful application of robotic technology in complex surgical procedures relies on appropriate mentorship to guide surgeons through a period of rapid innovation. The role of such mentors, and the roles of other members of the operating team such as trainees, nursing staff, and industry representatives, should be discussed in the context of principles of ethical surgical innovation as laid out by guidelines from organizations such as the Society of University Surgeons.

Conflict of Interest

Ethical scientific research should strive to be devoid of bias. One form of bias that has garnered much attention in the lay press has been the issue of conflict of interest [15], which can be defined in many ways. Commonly, it refers to a set of conditions in which professional judgment concerning a primary interest may be perceived to be unduly influencing a secondary interest [16]. Conflicts of interest may revolve around financial reimbursement, industry support of research, or – as previously mentioned – publication and promotion. It is important to understand that even the perception of a conflict of interest can damage the trust that the public, patient or subject has in the medical and research enterprise. Conflicts of interest that are handled poorly can also injure the surgeon-scientist's reputation and career. The surgeon-scientist must therefore be aware of any and all potential conflicts of interest when it comes to his/her research. In an era when surgeons frequently partner with industry in the conduct of research, it is not possible to eradicate all potential for conflict of interest. In fact, a conflict does not necessarily imply unethical behavior, but rather the potential to have bias influence the outcome of the study. As such, the ethical ramifications are determined more by the manner in which the surgeon-scientist handles and addresses any potential conflict of interest.

Full disclosure can mitigate some conflicts of interest. Academic institutions typically have a specific policy that outlines the rules of what and how potential conflicts of interest must be disclosed. It is each surgeon-scientist's responsibility to familiarize themselves with their respective institution's policy and ensure compliance with these policies. Researchers are ethically obliged to divulge connections between any third party and their research that may seem to benefit themselves or their research. Disclosure should include not only financial remuneration for the specific investigator, but in most circumstances any family members with financial ties. As it is often difficult for individual investigators to objectively assess the potential for personal conflict of interest, independent institutional verification and review is warranted. Most institutions focus on determining the degree to which a conflict of interest may be present and ensuring appropriate management of any conflicts identified. Some conflicts can be managed with external oversight to allow researchers to continue their work. In some circumstances, however, certain conflicts cannot be managed and researchers may need to divest from a specific area of research or the industry tie.

Publication and Authorship

Publication is the "coin" of the academic realm. Authorship – particularly primary or "first" author and "senior" author status – is important to the surgeon-scientist as it has implications for career advancement and promotion. Unfortunately, issues around authorship can be ethically problematic. Common issues include providing appropriate recognition for those who do the most work and avoiding the listing of those who may not have contributed in a meaningful way to the work. In one scenario, junior researchers can be denied first authorship despite having contributed significantly to the study (through study design, data collection, data analysis, drafting and/or revision of the article). At other times, authorship is "awarded" on an honorary or "quid pro quo" basis to senior individuals who have not had a meaningful contribution to the research project. In an effort to standardize criteria for authorship, the Vancouver Group has defined requirements for recognition as an author based on several criteria [17]. Authors should be involved in (a) the design of the experiment and/or the analysis and interpretation of the data, (b) drafting or critically revising the manuscript and (c) final approval of the product to be published. In essence, all manuscript authors need to have made substantial contributions to the work and be able to take responsibility for the work. Participation as a co-author based solely on seniority, funding, or collection of the data (e.g. the surgeon who solely operated on the cases being studied) does not constitute authorship.

Discussion about authorship is best done when the project is beginning. The principal investigator and junior researcher should have open, transparent, and frank conversations about expectations regarding the project. Specifically, the principal investigator should establish what his/her expectations are regarding the amount and type of work that is expected of the junior researcher if he/she is to be the first author. The junior researcher then has a much better idea of what will be required in order to claim primary authorship. In some instances, discussions about possible contingency plans should also be explored (e.g. "if you are unable to finish the project and the next researcher does most of the work, we will need to re-examine the issue of authorship"). As with most ethical dilemmas, the key to successfully navigating the waters of authorship is good communication and a relationship built on mutual respect and trust.

Special Considerations Regarding Quality Improvement Initiatives

The Accreditation Council for Graduate Medical Education and the American College of Surgeons now tasks all residency programs to ensure that graduates have experience in quality improvement processes and initiatives [18]. While this experience likely varies dramatically across the spectrum of surgical residencies, the goal of developing national leaders in quality improvement is clear. Importantly, however, the designation of a project as a quality improvement measure does not mitigate the need for ethical evaluation when patient care is impacted. In fact, the ethical questions that face researchers in other fields may be more difficult to answer for many studies completed under the auspices of quality improvement. Nevertheless, whenever data from human subjects is obtained in an effort to provide generalizable knowledge this is considered "human subjects research" and is subject to The Common Rule (as discussed earlier in this chapter).

In quality improvement research, the direct target of the intervention typically focuses on system processes, environment, or clinician behavior. The end-results, however, are routinely patient-centered outcomes. This raises questions that may be difficult to answer, such as actual "trickle-down" risk to patients, the relative benefits to patients, and the appropriate consent or disclosure method that should be entertained [19]. Even determining who should undergo consent, and if certain quality improvement projects are appropriate at all can be ethically challenging. The role of an IRB in approving quality improvement projects may also vary from the historical norm. Rather than an IRB insisting on rigorous methodology (such as randomization) and statistical planning (with well-defined primary outcome measures identified), often quality improvement initiatives are deemed to meet the federal definitions of minimal risk and undergo expedited ethical consideration. Surgeon-scientists must avoid, however, casually defining a research project as a quality initiative solely for the purposes of an expedited IRB review and remember that the ethical considerations for quality improvement work are likely just as important as "standard" research.

Special Considerations Regarding Basic Science Research in an Academic Environment

David Resnik has argued that there are several aspects of the research environment that may make it particularly susceptible to moral strain [20]. Researchers are pressured to publish papers, effectively utilize limited laboratory resources, and obtain funding. Unfortunately, occasionally a researcher may succumb to these pressures and begin to ignore ambiguous data, negative results, or begin to "massage" the data. The laboratory environment – not unlike surgical training itself – can often be hierarchical in nature, making some students or residents feel pressured to do things to "satisfy" the expectations of their supervisor. Power imbalances between the lead researcher and mentees may potentially affect how research is performed and how results are reported. Because positive results are often rewarded and negative results are frequently seen as failures, investigators may feel tempted to "fudge" the results. As most researchers can anticipate the "desired" or "correct" results, they may try to justify this behavior by telling themselves "I know this is how it really would have turned out if…." Dishonesty in scientific research, however, undermines the most fundamental ethical principles: trust, honesty, and validity.

Dishonesty includes fabrication, falsification, and plagiarism [21]. Whereas fabrication is the baseless creation of data in the absence of empirical experimental results, falsification is the manipulation or misrepresentation of data or results that were obtained from experiments. Misrepresentation most commonly involves the purposeful omission of findings that contradict the desired outcome. In data collection, this can include omission of certain data points to "tighten up" the data (e.g. "I am going to leave these three data points out because they are clearly 'outliers'"). In data analysis, this often includes guided manipulation of the data (e.g. "torturing" the data with statistics to get a desired or anticipated result). Finally, the most overt form of dishonesty is plagiarism, which is the wholesale appropriation of another researcher's ideas, work, or written word as your own. Plagiarism can include the reproduction of another researcher's ideas at a meeting or the reproduction of another researcher's written word in publication. Plagiarism is a serious infraction of research ethics and can have long-term negative implications for a researcher's career. As such, investigators should take particular effort to give credit where it is due and fastidiously avoid reproducing the work of others. All forms of dishonesty seriously undermine and erode the integrity of scientific research and therefore should be avoided at all costs.

The hallmark of good, ethical laboratory research also includes a commitment to an open research environment and a dedication to meticulous methodology. An open research environment can help cultivate the scientific process by allowing ambiguous or "wrong" results to be discussed and examined. Errors can be quickly identified in a non-punitive manner and corrective measures can be implemented expeditiously. Negative results can also be openly accepted and research efforts can be directed towards novel ideas or solutions. Mentors and research leaders are therefore ethically obligated to help foster open communication in the research setting. Mentors should interact with mentees not only to exchange research ideas but also to model good scientific standards and ethical research behavior. It is imperative that scientists avoid careless research as it is fundamentally unethical. In addition to wasting societal resources, it also exposes subjects (e.g. humans and/or animals) to unnecessary risks, and may result in erroneous findings that can damage future research endeavors or even injure patients. As such, researchers need to exercise caution in their research to identify and obviate "avoidable" errors. The standard of triple-checking key findings should be regarded as a minimum requirement for the ethical conduct of research. While at times this may delay the desire to produce results quickly, it may prevent the propagation of technical errors of experimentation or unconscious bias from finding their way to published conclusions. While some errors are honest mistakes, the ethical surgeon-scientist strives to avoid errors in their research as a means to respect the scientific process, as well as the resources entrusted to him/her.

Conclusion

Surgeon-scientists are frequently faced with ethical challenges both at the bedside and in the laboratory. The research environment is enmeshed with issues requiring objectivity, honesty, and respect for persons. Seniority, hierarchy, and power imbalances can further complicate the ethical landscape of the surgeon-scientist. An environment characterized by open communication, high ethical standards, and a focus on doing "what is right" should be the goal of each surgeon-scientist. To be a scientist is to engage in behavior with certain moral and ethical implications [22]. Surgeons should not shrink from this responsibility. Instead, academic surgeons should actively engage in the moral issues inextricably linked to their research. It is only through this engagement that we are empowered to not only be better researchers, but also to be better physicians, improving the quality of care we deliver to those who depend on us for help.

References

1. Markel H. Experiments and observations: how William Beaumont and Alexis St. Martin seized the moment of scientific progress. JAMA. 2009;302(7):804–6.
2. Fost N, Levine RJ. The dysregulation of human subjects research. JAMA. 2007;298(18):2196–8.
3. Nuremberg Military Tribunal. The nuremberg code. JAMA. 1996;276(20):1691.
4. World Medical Association declaration of Helsinki. Recommendations guiding physicians in biomedical research involving human subjects. JAMA. 1997;277(11):925–6.
5. McCallum JM, Arekere DM, Green BL, et al. Awareness and knowledge of the U.S. Public Health Service syphilis study at Tuskegee: implications for biomedical research. J Health Care Poor Underserved. 2006;17(4):716–33.
6. Goliszek A. In the name of science. New York: St. Martin's Press; 2003.
7. Services UDoHaH. Protections of human subjects, 45 CFR 46. 1991.
8. Skolnick BE. Ethical and institutional review board issues. Adv Neurol. 1998;76:253–62.
9. Weijer C, Dickens B, Meslin EM. Bioethics for clinicians: 10. Research ethics. CMAJ. 1997;156(8):1153–7.
10. Emanuel EJ, Wendler D, Grady C. What makes clinical research ethical? JAMA. 2000;283(20):2701–11.
11. McKneally MF, Ignagni E, Martin DK, D'Cruz J. The leap to trust: perspective of cholecystectomy patients on informed decision making and consent. J Am Coll Surg. 2004;199(1):51–7.
12. Biffl WL, Spain DA, Reitsma AM, et al. Responsible development and application of surgical innovations: a position statement of the Society of University Surgeons. J Am Coll Surg. 2008;206(3):1204–9.
13. Jones JW. Ethics of rapid surgical technological advancement. Ann Thorac Surg. 2000;69(3):676–7.
14. Larson JA, Johnson MH, Bhayani SB. Application of surgical safety standards to robotic surgery: five principles of ethics for nonmaleficence. J Am Coll Surg. 2014;218(2):290–3.
15. Morin K, Rakatansky H, Riddick Jr FA, et al. Managing conflicts of interest in the conduct of clinical trials. JAMA. 2002;287(1):78–84.
16. Thompson DF. Understanding financial conflicts of interest. N Engl J Med. 1993;329(8):573–6.
17. Uniform requirements for manuscripts submitted to biomedical journals. International Committee of Medical Journal Editors. JAMA. 1993;269(17):2282–6.
18. Accreditation Council for Graduate Medical Education. ACGME common program requirements [Internet]. 2015 [Cited 30 May 2016]. Available from: http://www.acgme.org/Portals/0/PFAssets/ProgramRequirements/CPRs_07012015.pdf.
19. Sugarman J, Califf RM. Ethics and regulatory complexities for pragmatic clinical trials. JAMA. 2014;331(23):2381–2.
20. Resnik D. The ethics of science: an introduction. New York: Routledge; 1998.
21. National Academy of Sciences NAoE, Institute of Medicine. Responsible science: ensuring the integrity of the research process. Washington, DC: National Academy Press; 1992.
22. Pawlik TM, Platteborze N, Souba WW. Ethics and surgical research: what should guide our behavior? J Surg Res. 1999;87(2):263–9.

Chapter 5
Study Design and Analysis in Clinical Research

Hemalkumar B. Mehta and Taylor S. Riall

This chapter serves an introduction to study design and data analysis for surgeons undertaking observational research. It is not intended to provide an in-depth review of all possible biostatistical methods. Rather, it is designed to assist surgeons in critically reviewing the literature and becoming informed users of biostatistics. The chapter will cover both study design and analysis, as the final product in any study is critically dependent on both factors. If a study is poorly designed, no amount of statistical analysis will compensate. Likewise, a well-designed study can produce irrelevant results if it is not properly analyzed. We encourage surgeons to consult with a statistician throughout the course of their study, from design to publication, in order to prevent critical errors in study design and data analysis. We also recommend formal training in basic biostatistics for surgeon-scientists. This allows you to do your own basic data analysis and enables the use of your clinical knowledge to guide the statistician in designing your study and interpreting your data to get clinically meaningful results.

The goal of the chapter is to address major concepts in data analysis providing the reader a foundation for analyzing and interpreting data applicable to clinical research. It will provide a framework in which surgeons can interpret the literature, evaluate and review scientific articles, and evaluate study protocols, including identification of strengths and weaknesses of the study design and analysis, as well as potential errors. This information can then be used to analyze and interpret your own data or the data of others, communicate the results clearly, and apply the results to patient care.

H.B. Mehta, Ph.D.
Department of Surgery, University of Texas Medical Branch,
Galveston, TX 77555-0541, USA

T.S. Riall, M.D., Ph.D. (✉)
Department of Surgery, University of Arizona,
Tucson, AZ 85658, USA

Study Design

In order to understand the conclusions that can be drawn from a study, it is critical to understand the study design. In medicine, study designs fall into two broad categories: (1) observational studies in which subjects are observed and their outcomes documented without allocation of treatment, and (2) experimental studies in which investigators allocate the treatment. In addition, research studies can be prospective or retrospective. A cohort is a group of patients with something in common who will remain part of that group over time. In prospective studies the direction of inquiry is forward from the cohort inception, and events occur after the study begins. In retrospective studies, the events have happened before the study begins, and the direction of the inquiry is backward in time.

There are four types of observational studies: (1) case reports or case-series, (2) cross-sectional studies, (3) case-control studies, and (4) cohort studies. Case-series studies are simple descriptive accounts of interesting characteristics in a group of patients. Such studies do not include control patients who do not have the disease or condition being described. These studies often serve as the foundation for future case-control and cohort studies. For example, when introducing a new procedure such as single-incision laparoscopic cholecystectomy, one might want to report the outcomes of the first group of patients undergoing the procedure to demonstrate safety and feasibility. This may then lead to case-control and cohort studies comparing it to the current gold standard – in this case, standard four-incision laparoscopic cholecystectomy.

Cross-sectional studies include surveys, polls, and prevalence studies. They analyze data collected on a group of subjects at a single point in time. The intent of a cross-sectional study is to provide a description of what is happening at that single time point. Cross-sectional studies can provide prevalence of a condition (the number of people with the condition divided by the total population at one point in time). Incidence, or the number of people who develop a condition over a specified period of time, cannot be ascertained in cross-sectional studies. Cross-sectional studies cannot be used to determine causation or estimate treatment effect.

Case-control and cohort studies are often termed longitudinal studies, where subjects are followed over time. The primary difference between the two study types is the direction of the inquiry. Case-control studies are retrospective. The "cases" are selected based on the presence of some disease or outcome, while "controls" are individuals without the disease or outcome. For example, you might want to study the effect of clopidogrel on bleeding risk in emergent surgical procedures. The outcome, bleeding, is relatively rare. In a case-control study, the cases are patients undergoing emergent surgery who had a postoperative bleeding event and the controls were patients undergoing emergent surgery who did not have a bleeding event. You then look back and compare the effect of the exposure (clopidogrel) on bleeding events in the cases and controls. Case-control studies are efficient for unusual conditions or outcomes and are relatively easy to perform, but it can often be difficult to identify an appropriate control. In addition, high-quality medical records are essential. Such studies are especially susceptible to selection and detection bias. The results of case-control studies are often presented as odds ratios (OR).

Traditional cohort studies are prospective. Retrospective cohort studies are studies in which the cohort is identified based on historical medical records and the follow-up period is partly or completely in the past. Cohort studies are optimal for studying the incidence, course, and risk factors for a disease since subjects are followed over time. Using the same example with a cohort study design, the investigator would define the cohort as patients undergoing emergent surgical procedures (all at risk for developing postoperative bleeding events). All potential risk factors are assessed at the onset of the study (before surgery). Patients are then followed prospectively to observe the effect of exposure of interest (clopidogrel) and all other covariates or potential confounders are controlled for in the analysis. The results of a cohort study are usually presented as relative risk. Prospective cohort studies minimize selection, information, recall, and measurement bias discussed below. They often require a long time for completion and are not good for looking at rare outcomes.

In experimental studies, subjects are allocated to specific treatment groups. These studies involve the use of controls that can be concurrent, sequential (cross-over design), or historical. Randomized clinical trials (RCTs) are considered the gold standard. Rigorous randomization and large sample sizes minimize or eliminate errors due to confounding, bias, and chance. Disadvantages of RCTs include significant time and expense, narrow cohort selection which limits generalizability, and difficulty accruing patients. In clinical medicine and surgery especially it is not always possible to conduct RCTs. They require equality of treatment options in the clinician's judgment, significant resources, and reasonable expectation of patient accrual.

Sources of Error in Medical Research

All research is susceptible to invalid conclusions from confounding, bias, and chance. A confounder is a variable that is associated with both the predictor (or independent variable) and the outcome of interest (or dependent variable). The confounder or risk factor may not be evenly distributed between the control and study groups and can lead to a spurious association between the predictor and the outcome of interest. Common confounders include gender, age, socioeconomic status, and comorbidities. For example, if you study the relationship between coffee drinking and pancreatic cancer, you might find an association (Fig. 5.1). However, this association may be entirely explained by smoking status, a known risk factor for pancreatic cancer. If more coffee drinkers than controls are smokers, you will identify an incorrect association between coffee drinking and smoking if you do not control for smoking. It is critical to control for confounding, especially in observational studies.

Bias is non-random, systematic error in the design or conduct of a study. Bias is often unintentional and there are many types. The types of bias and examples are

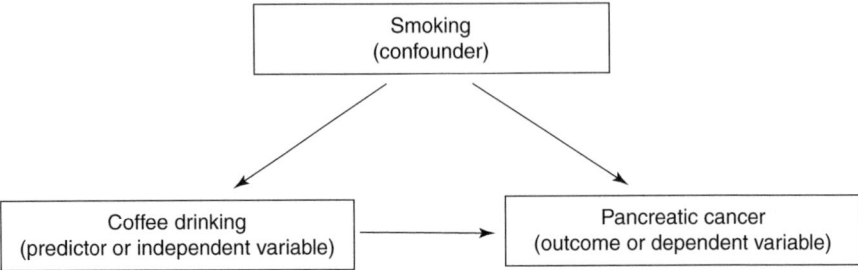

Fig. 5.1 Confounding. In this example, smoking acts as a confounder. Smoking is associated with both coffee drinking (the factor being studied) and developing pancreatic cancer (outcome). If more coffee drinkers than controls are smokers, you will identify an incorrect association between coffee drinking and smoking if you do no control for smoking

summarized in Table 5.1. It should be noted that bias can also occur if "bad" data are arbitrarily rejected. The effects of bias and confounding can be minimized by good study design. Experimental designs minimize bias. Randomization minimizes selection bias and, theoretically, equally distributes measured as well as unmeasured confounders. Matching, propensity score analysis, and instrumental variable analysis can help decrease bias in observational studies, especially when exposure or receipt of treatment is not randomized.

Inferential Statistics

All studies are based on a sample and make inferences about the truth in the overall population of interest. A statistical hypothesis is a statement of belief about population parameters. The purpose of hypothesis testing is to permit generalizations from a sample to the population from which it came. Hypothesis testing confirms or refutes the assertion that the observed findings in a study occurred by chance alone. The null hypothesis, symbolized by H_0 is a statement claiming there is no difference between the observed findings and the population. In other words, if the null hypothesis is true, the finding likely occurred by chance alone. The alternative hypothesis, H_1, is that the there is an association, or that the finding did not occur by chance alone.

By constructing a 2×2 table (Table 5.2), we can evaluate the possible outcomes of study. Statistical inferences are subject to two types of errors. Type I errors or alpha (α) errors occur when a significant association is found when there is no true association. By convention, most statistical analyses set α at 0.05, which means that if we reject the null hypothesis (confirm an association) there is less than a 5% chance that the findings occurred by chance alone. The P-value is a measure of the probability of a type I error. If the P-value is less than α, then we reject the null hypothesis and conclude the result is significant. The P-value is an arbitrary cutoff point and gives no information about the strength of the association, only the probability that the outcome did not occur by chance. A P-value may be statistically

5 Study Design and Analysis in Clinical Research

Table 5.1 Types of bias

Type of bias	Description	Example
Sampling bias	Occurs when data are obtained from a non-random sample of the population.	Selecting patients from a single town; this is not representative of general population
Selection bias	Occurs when treatment assignments are made on the basis of certain characteristics of the patients such that the two groups are not similar	Cancer patients with no comorbidities are more likely to undergo active treatment versus patients with several comorbidities are less likely to get treatment
Prevalence or incidence bias	Occurs when a condition is characterized by early fatalities	Protective effect of smoking on Alzheimer's disease (AD) can be explained due to the fact smokers die early and don't develop AD versus non-smokers live longer and develop AD
Membership bias	Occurs because one or more of the characteristics that cause people to belong to groups are related to the outcome of interest	Membership in a group that may differ systematically from the general population
Protopathic bias	Occurs if a particular treatment or exposure was started, stopped, or otherwise changed because of the baseline manifestation caused by a disease or other outcome event	Treatment of postmenopausal syndrome with estrogen may lead to a false association between estrogen replacement and endometrial cancer
Immortal time bias	Occurs because death or study outcome cannot happen in certain time period because the way study is designed or analyzed	Patients who died waiting for cardiac transplantations were classified in non-transplant group. Thus, artificially showing higher survival benefits of cardiac transplant
Information bias	Occurs because of misclassification of the risk factor being assessed and/or misclassification of the disease or other outcome itself. It is a type of bias that occurs when measurement of information (e.g., exposure or outcome) differs among study groups	Patients with exposure followed for a longer period of time compared to patients without exposure
Non-responder bias	Occurs when subjects fail to respond to a survey; responders often have different characteristics than non-responders	Patients with disease are more likely to respond to the survey compared to patients without disease
Recall bias	Occurs when patients are asked to recall certain events; people in a group with an adverse outcome are more likely to remember certain events	Women with breast cancer provide complete and accurate description of exposure to oral contraceptives compared to women without breast cancer

(continued)

Table 5.1 (continued)

Type of bias	Description	Example
Detection bias	Occurs when a new diagnostic technique is introduced that is capable of detecting a disease at an earlier stage	Women taking postmenopausal hormonal supplements are likely to see their doctors more often than other women, therefore more likely to be examined for breast cancer
Interviewer bias	Occurs when the opinion or prejudice on the part of an interviewer is displayed during the interview process and affects the outcome of the interview	Interviewer may ask more probing questions to patients with disease than patients without disease

Table 5.2 Hypothesis testing

	True population results	
Experimental results	No association	Association
No Association	Correct	β or type II error[a]
Association	α or type I error[b]	Correct

[a]Power = $1 - \beta$ where β is the probability of a type II error
[b]P-value is equal to the probability of a type I error

significant but clinically irrelevant, which is common in very large studies that are often overpowered for the outcome being measured. The use of confidence intervals instead of P-values has become increasingly common, as these intervals convey information about the clinical significance, the magnitude of the differences, and the precision of the measurement. When comparing two groups, 95 % confidence intervals are most commonly used; if these intervals do not overlap, they are considered statistically different. Wide confidence intervals indicate lack of precision in the measurement.

When a study demonstrates no significant association, the potential error of concern is a type II or beta (β) error. Type II errors are expressed as power. The power of a study is the probability of finding a significant association if one truly exists. Power is defined as 1 – probability of a type II error (β). Acceptable power is usually set at greater than or equal to 80 %. Power is directly related to sample size. There are four elements in a power analysis: α, β, effect size, and sample size. The effect size is the difference that you want or expect to be able to detect between two groups. For the previously used example of the effect of clopidogrel on bleeding risk, you need to know the expected rate of bleeding events and the expected increase in bleeding events associated with clopidogrel. Power increases with increasing sample size and increasing effect size. We caution against choosing an effect size that is clinically irrelevant in order to make the power over 80 %; effect size should be based on the literature and clinical expertise, and sample size should follow, not vice versa. You should work with your statistician before you begin a study to ensure that you will realistically be able to accrue enough patients to generate sufficient power to answer your question.

Types of Variables

Patient characteristics can be measured on various scales using different types of variables. The variable type determines the statistical methodology. Broadly speaking, data can be categorical (qualitative) or numerical (quantitative). Within categorical data, variables can be either nominal or ordinal. Nominal variables have two or more categories. Examples include sex, race, the presence or absence of a condition (i.e., congestive heart failure) or dichotomous outcomes (yes or no). Ordinal data follows a specific order. A classic example would be tumor staging, i.e., stage I to stage IV. Numerical scales are used for quantitative observations. These can be discrete or continuous. A continuous scale, such as age, duration of survival, or operative time, has numbers on a continuum. A discrete scale consists of data that can take on integer values only. Examples are counts such as the number of hospital admissions, number of previous operations, or number of falls.

Descriptive Statistics and Comparison of Groups

Measures of Central Tendency

Numeric data can be summarized by measures of central tendency such as mean, median, and mode, and in terms of measures of spread or dispersion, such as range, standard deviation, and interquartile range. The most common measure of central tendency is the mean. It is the sum of the observations divided by the number of observations. The mean is sensitive to extreme outlying values, especially when the sample size is small. The median is the middle observation, where half the observations are smaller and half are bigger. If there is an even number of observations, the median is the mean of the two middle values. The median is less sensitive to extreme values than the mean. We often use median values to describe survival. Telling someone the median survival is 18 months after a curative-intent operation for pancreatic cancer means that half the people who have such an operation will survive that long. The mode is the value that occurs the most frequently, commonly used for large numbers of observations. If a dataset has two modes, it is called bimodal.

When determining which measure of central tendency is best, you need to consider the scale of the measurement and the shape of the distribution of observations (Fig. 5.2). If observations are evenly distributed around the mean, the mean is equal to the median and the distribution is symmetric (Fig. 5.2a). If outlying observations are all large, the mean will be larger than the median and the distribution will be skewed to the right (positively skewed, Fig. 5.2b). If they are all small, the distribution mean will be lower than the median and the distribution will be skewed to the left (negatively skewed, Fig. 5.2c). The mean should be used for numerical data that are not skewed. The median can be used for numerical data with a skewed distribution. The mode is useful for bimodal distributions. For example, there is a bimodal

Fig. 5.2 Commonly seen distributions of observations in clinical studies. (**a**) Normal distribution. The mean is equal to the median. (**b**) Positively skewed or skewed to the right. The mean is greater than the median due to large outlying observations. (**c**) Negatively skewed or skewed to the left. The mean is less than the median due to small outlying observations

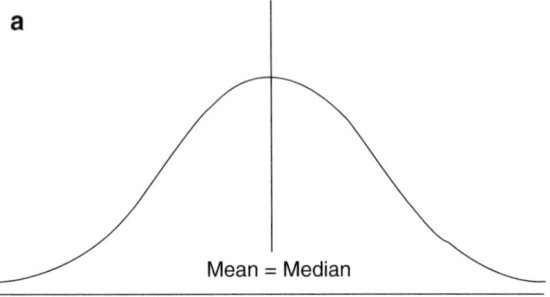
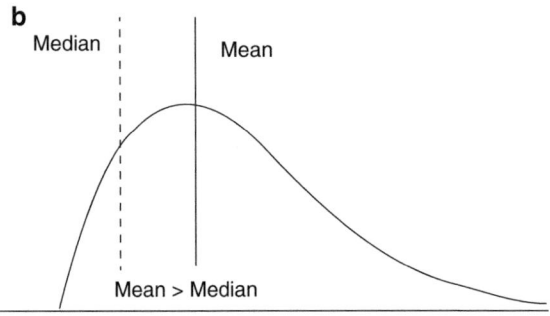
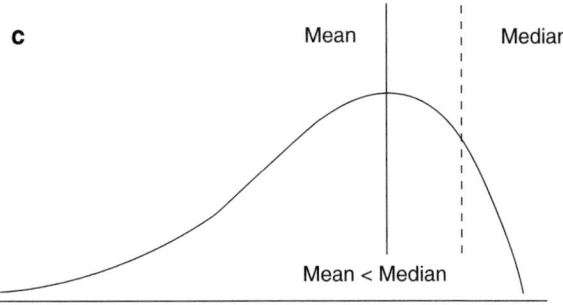

distribution for incidence of Crohn's disease occurring most commonly in patients in their teens/twenties and patients in their sixties. For this type of distribution the mean is not useful or descriptive.

Measures of Spread

While the mean provides useful information, the spread (dispersion or variation) of the observations around the mean provides more information. The range is the difference between the smallest and largest observation. It is common to give maximum and minimum values, which are more useful than the range. The range is used to emphasize extreme values.

Standard deviation (SD) is the most commonly used measure of variation in medicine. It describes how observations cluster around the mean and it is the basis for many statistical tests used to compare means between groups. For each observation, the deviation from the mean is calculated and squared. The sum of the squared deviations for all observations is divided by the number of observations minus one. This value is called the variance. The square root of the variance is the SD. Regardless of the distribution of the data, at least 75 % of observations fall between the mean plus or minus two SDs. If a distribution is bell-shaped or normal, it has special characteristics; 67 % of observations in a normal distribution lie between the mean ± 1 SD, 95 % lie between the mean ± 2 SD, and 99.7 % lie between the mean ± 3 SD. If the mean is smaller than two standard deviations, the data are probably skewed. SD is used when the mean is used and is best when the data are symmetric.

A percentile is the percentage of distribution that is at or below a particular number. Percentiles are commonly used to determine the "normal" ranges of laboratory values. Values lower than the 2.5 percentile and higher than the 97.5 percentile (greater or less than 2 SD from the mean) are considered abnormal. The interquartile range is the difference between the 25th and 75th percentile (or first and third quartiles), or the central 50 % of observations. Percentiles and interquartile ranges are used when the median is used for skewed data or when the mean is used but the goal is to compare individual observations with a set of norms. Box plots provide visual representation of a continuous variable by showing minimum value, maximum value, median and interquartile range in a single figure (Fig. 5.3a). Histograms are used to show the distribution of a continuous variable (Fig. 5.3b). Stem-and-leaf plots, dot plots, and scatter plots are also used to visualize continuous data. Looking at data visually is helpful to identify outliers, and it gives sense of distribution of the data.

Comparison of Numeric Variables

Univariate analysis is used to assess the relationship of a single independent variable (predictor) and a single dependent variable (outcome). Statistical tests for comparing means of continuous variables that are normally distributed include the Student's t test for two independent groups and the paired t test for paired samples. If the continuous variable is not normally distributed, non-parametric tests are used. These tests include the Wilcoxon rank sum test (also known as the Mann–Whitney U test) for two independent groups and the Wilcoxon signed-rank test for paired samples. Analysis of variance (ANOVA) is used to compare means among three or more normally distributed, independent groups. When comparing three or more groups, the P-value (corresponding to an F test) indicates an overall significant difference and not differences between any two groups. To determine differences between any two groups you need to do post-hoc comparison tests to perform multiple, pairwise comparisons including Tukey, Bonferroni, Newman-Keuls, and Fisher. The Kruskal-Wallis test is used to compare medians for three more independent groups in which the means are not normally distributed.

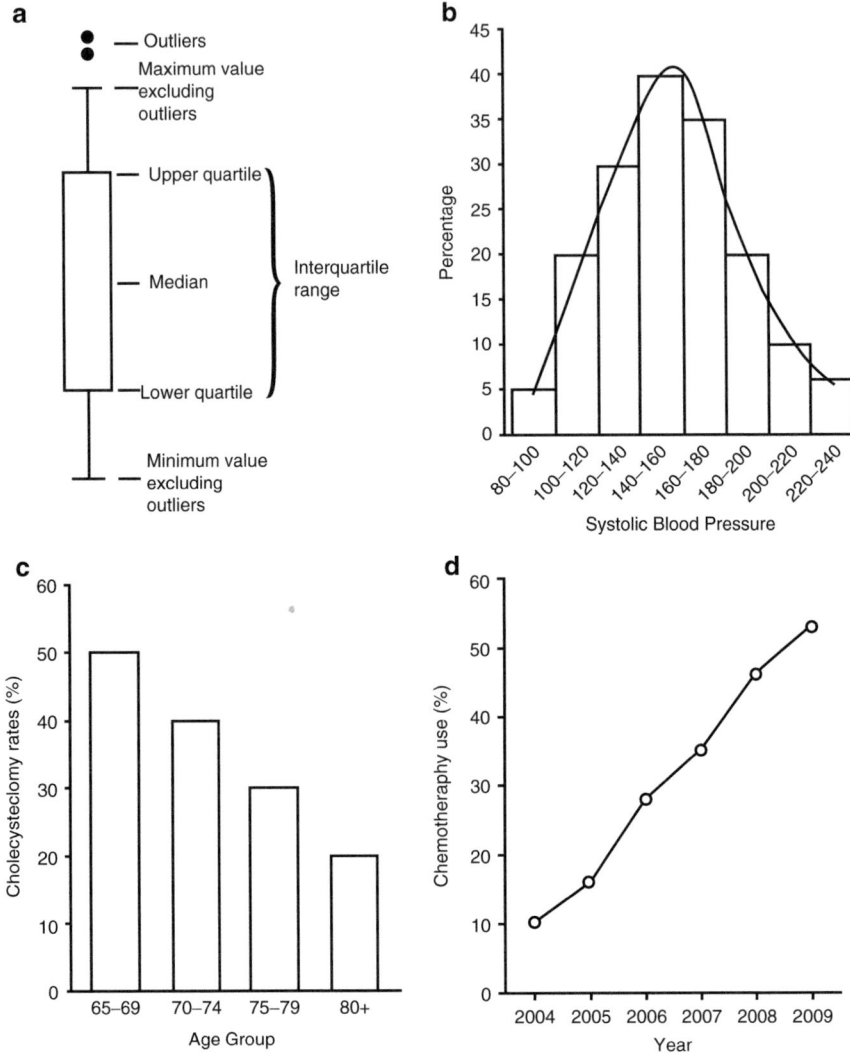

Fig. 5.3 (**a**) Box plot. (**b**) Histogram of systolic blood pressure. (**c**) Bar chart showing cholecystectomy rates by different age group. (**d**) Line chart showing increase in chemotherapy rates by year

Comparison of Categorical Values

Categorical variables are expressed as proportions and can be demonstrated in 2×2 tables for two independent groups up to $n \times n$ tables for n independent groups. The one- and two-way frequency tables are often used to summarize results and describe a cohort. One-way frequency table lists results for one variable whereas two-way tables form cross-tabulation of two variables. Two-way tables often include P-values comparing the frequencies of different variables between groups using appropriate inferential statistics. Bar charts provide visualization of the data that can also be displayed in a tabular format (Fig. 5.3c). Chi-square tests are used to compare proportions for categorical or ordinal values with two or more independent groups. In the case of more than two groups, the resulting P-value indicates the overall difference between the groups but does not provide pairwise comparisons. When expected cell frequencies are less than five, Fisher exact tests should be used. For matched samples, the McNemar test is used for two variables and the Cochran Q test for three or more. Line graphs can be used to show the value of a variable over time (Fig. 5.3d). The increase or decrease in the trend can be tested statistically using Cochran-Armitage trend test.

Observational Studies and Analysis of Secondary Data

Health services or outcomes research often involves secondary data analysis of large administrative datasets that were not initially collected for research purposes. These datasets include Medicare data; Surveillance, Epidemiology, and End Results (SEER) tumor registry data; hospital discharge data; tumor registries; the National Cancer Data Bank; and the Nationwide Inpatient Sample. The American College of Surgeons-National Surgical Quality Improvement Program (ACS-NSQIP) public use file is collected for research purposes and uses clinical, not administrative data, but has similar limitations in that treatment is not randomized.

As administrative data do not measure specific clinical outcomes, the investigator is dependent on surrogate measures, usually in the form of diagnosis codes, to identify specific clinical conditions. You must carefully consider how you will measure exposure and outcomes using these surrogate measures keeping in mind that certain events and diagnoses are more accurately coded than others. For example, major surgical procedures (source of income) are accurately billed, whereas covariates or exposures such as smoking that do not generate revenue, are much less accurately coded.

The use of such data is complex and poses many analytical difficulties. It is absolutely critical to understand if the particular dataset can actually answer your question. For example, you might want to use SEER tumor registry data to evaluate several published algorithms for predicting additional axillary node positivity in patients with a positive sentinel lymph node biopsy. You need to carefully look through the documentation. SEER collected information on sentinel lymph node biopsy after 2002. However, they give only the final nodal status of the axilla and you are unable to separate the status of the sentinel nodes from the status of the remainder of the axilla, so you cannot do the study.

In addition, the coding in administrative datasets changes over time. For example, new diagnosis and procedure codes are added and staging schemes are altered and it is easy to make errors. This will be a major challenge for health services investigators as we switch from the International Classification of Diseases, Clinical Modification (ICD-CM)-9 to ICD-CM-10. We recommend working with someone who has used the dataset before. Download all the relevant coding manuals and information from associated websites and be sure you understand changes in coding schemes over time. Finally, the manipulation of these datasets requires significant expertise in data management and should not be performed without the help of an experienced data manager/biostatistician.

Administrative data are observational. As such, they are susceptible to significant confounding and selection bias. This often requires advanced statistical techniques to overcome the inherent selection bias and there may be situations in which we cannot overcome this bias at all. In the next section, we discuss commonly used statistical methods to analyze observational data.

The Advanced Statistical Methods for Observational Data

Before you jump to complex statistical methods you need to understand your data by performing simple descriptive statistics including the frequencies of categorical variables, means, medians, distributions of continuous data, and univariate comparisons between groups. You then need to consult with a statistician. You must make sure you are using correct statistical methods, understand the assumptions of the statistical methods you are using, and make sure you do not violate the assumptions.

Multivariable Analysis

Multivariable analysis is a method of obtaining a mathematical relationship between an outcome variable (dependent variable) and multiple predictor variables (independent variables). Various forms of regression are commonly used to control for confounding and establish independent associations among predictor variables and outcomes. Multiple regression fits data into a model that defines the outcome (Y) as a function of multiple predictor variables ($x_1, x_2, \ldots, x_j$) and the regression equation takes many forms depending on whether the outcome variable is continuous, categorical or time-to-event. Its general form is: $Y = \beta_0 + \beta_1 x_1 + \beta_2 x_2 + \ldots + \beta_j x_j$, where Y is the outcome, x_1 through x_j are the covariates (predictors), β_0 is the intercept, and β_1 through β_j are coefficients describing the effect of the specific covariate on the outcome. The independent variables in any multivariable regression can be either continuous or categorical. This methodology can be used to evaluate factors associated with a specific outcomes or control for known confounders when evaluating a specific relationship between a predictor and outcome.

Linear Regression Analysis

Linear regression is used to study the relationship of a continuous outcome variable to a single predictor variable. In an example given by Afifi et al. in Computer-Aided Multivariate Analysis (see selected references), the researcher is evaluating the effect of height on forced expiratory volume (FEV1). The basic regression equation is: FEV1 = $\beta_0 + \beta_1$(height in inches). The relationship discovered was FEV1 = −4.087 + 0.118 (height in inches). So for each inch of increased height, FEV1 increases by a factor of 0.118.

However, we know that other factors such as age also affect FEV1. Multiple linear regression allows these variables to be added to the model providing a less biased estimate. When age is added to the model the result is FEV1 = −2.761 − 0.027 (age) + 0.114 (height). After controlling for age, the FEV1 increases 0.114 with inch increase in height.

Logistic Regression Analysis

Logistic regression is commonly used when an outcome variable is dichotomous (yes/no). Logistic regression models the log of the odds of the outcome variable. The equation is in the form: Logit $[p] = \beta_0 + \beta_1 x_1 + \beta_2 x_2 + \ldots + \beta_j x_j$. In this case, odds ratios for each factor can be obtained by exponentiating the beta coefficient: Odds Ratio (OR) = e^β. If the OR is equal to one or the 95 % confidence interval includes 1, the associated predictor variable does not have a statistically significant association with the outcome variable. The 95 % CI is more informative than the p-value as it reflects the uncertainty around the point estimate, with a large CI meaning high uncertainty.

In a hypothetical example, the OR for surgical mortality (yes or no) in open compared to laparoscopic surgery may be 1.50 (95 % CI, 1.20–1.70) after controlling for confounders such as body mass index, comorbidities, operative procedure, etc. This can be interpreted as patients undergoing open surgery have a 50 % higher odds of operative mortality compared to patients undergoing laparoscopic surgery. The 95 % confidence interval indicates the uncertainty around the OR and it can be interpreted as increased odds of death can be as low as 20 % and as high as 70 %.

When constructing a regression model, you can start by putting all the factors in your conceptual model and eliminate factors that are not significant in stepwise fashion based on statistical tests (hypothesis is that $\beta = 0$, or the OR = 1). Conversely, you can start with only your relationship of interest (simple regression) and add factors in stepwise fashion. Your model should be based on your conceptual model. Some factors, while not significant, might be known confounders and should be forced into the model (not removed even if not significant).

Time-to-Event Analysis

Time-to-event analyses are used when the time to a specific event and not only the occurrence of the event is important. Survival analysis is the most common example. It is not enough to know if a patient died, but how long they lived before the event occurred, as there is a big difference between dying 1 month or 10 years after cancer surgery. The end point of a time-to-event analysis can be any endpoint such as readmission to the hospital, death, reoperation, etc. The Kaplan-Meier product limit method allows patients to enter the cohort at different points in time and have variable follow-up. This method is used when the exact date of an endpoint is known and event-free survival is calculated at each time point where an event occurs. Once the event occurs, the time from onset of the study to the event is recorded. A patient is censored if the event of interest does not occur during the follow-up period.

In a Kaplan-Meier survival analysis, a "survival" curve (time without an event) can be plotted to illustrate the percentage of patients event-free on the y-axis and follow-up time on the x-axis. While Kaplan-Meier curve plots survival probability at each time point, cumulative incidence curve plots failure (1-survival) probability. Cumulative incidence curve should be used in the presence of competing risk. For example, deaths due to non-cancer cause become a competing risk when the outcome of interest is cancer-specific deaths. Cox proportional hazards models are multivariable models using time-to-event information and allow for determination of independent predictors of a time-dependent outcome. The Cox model provides hazards ratio (HR); the interpretation of HR is the same as odds ratios.

Different statistical software such as SAS, STATA, SPSS, or R can be used to conduct basic and advanced data analysis.

Advanced Methods for Controlling for Selection Bias

Multilevel Modeling (MLM)

Multilevel modeling is also referred as hierarchical models, random effects models, and mixed effects models. Multilevel modeling can be used with linear, logistic or survival outcomes. The basic assumption of traditional regression method is that observations are sampled randomly from the population. However, this assumption may not hold while evaluating surgical outcomes. For example, patients who are operated by a same surgeon or in a same hospital are no longer independent because they are clustered within a surgeon or a hospital. In such scenario, outcomes for patients operated by the same surgeon or in the same hospital would be relatively similar.

Using traditional regression methods in such settings can violate the random sampling assumption and provide biased treatment effect. Multilevel models account for the clustering of patients within higher level. For example, patients (level 1) clustered within surgeons (level 2) represents a two-level model; patients (level 1) clustered within surgeons (level 2), and surgeons (level 2) clustered within hospitals (level 3) represents a three-level model. Patient, surgeon, and hospital level characteristics associated with exposure and the outcome should be included in the multilevel model. Model specifications and interpretation remains same as traditional regression analysis. Multilevel modeling can also be used to better understand the observed variation in health care practices. (See selected reference by Sheffield et al. [10])

Propensity Score (PS) Analysis

The propensity score analysis is an increasingly popular method to control selection bias and confounding by indication in observational studies. Propensity score analysis is appealing because it balances the treated and untreated groups across observable patient characteristics and acts as a pseudo-randomized controlled design. Propensity score is particularly useful when outcome is rare and exposure is common. Propensity score analysis involves two-step approach. The first step involves the estimation of the propensity score and the second step involves use of propensity score to estimate treatment effect. Propensity score analysis can be used with linear, logistic or survival outcomes. The propensity score is defined as the probability of receiving treatment obtained from observed baseline patient characteristics. The usual approach to estimate propensity score is with logistic regression model. All variables that are associated with treatment and outcome (confounders), and are associated with outcome should be included as independent variables in the propensity score model. The second step involves use of propensity score to estimate the treatment effect. There are four available techniques including matching, regression adjustment, stratification, and weighting. The most common technique is propensity score matching because it is intuitive and works as pseudo-randomization. In this technique, patients who receive the treatment are matched with patients who did not receive the treatment based on their propensity scores, and analysis is performed on the matched sample.

Instrumental Variable (IV) Analysis

Instrumental variable (IV) analysis is a sophisticated method to help control for selection bias and unmeasured confounding in observational studies. It is appropriate when potential confounding variables are either unknown or difficult to measure. The primary assumption of most methods for estimating treatment effect using observational data is there is no unmeasured confounder. However, this assumption cannot be directly verified and one can argue on a substantive ground that some important variables may be missing, leading to bias in estimating treatment effect. The most critical element of an IV analysis is the instrumental variable itself. An IV is a measurable event or characteristic that gets a patient into a treatment group, but is not associated with the outcome directly or indirectly through unmeasured variables pathways. The difficulty in using IV analysis is in identifying an instrumental variable which meets the IV analysis assumptions: (1) an IV should be associated with treatment; (2) an IV should be unrelated to patient characteristics; and (3) an IV should be related to the outcome only through its association with treatment. Weak instruments may lead to larger standard errors and biased treatment effect. The choice of an instrument variable should be based on a well-thought-out conceptual framework. Some commonly used instrumental variables in health services research includes distance to the healthcare provider, physician or surgeon preference, regional variation, day of the week of hospital admission, calendar time, and drug co-payment amount. Results from a well-conducted IV analysis can provide an unbiased estimate of treatment effect, which is comparable to results obtained from a randomized controlled trial.

Difference-in-Difference Analysis

Observational studies are often used to study policy questions such as the effectiveness of policy change or policy implementation on improving outcomes. The difference-in-difference analysis is a commonly used technique to study effectiveness of policy level questions. (See selected reference by Dimick et al and Jha et al.) In the study by Jha et al., the research question was to evaluate the effect of pay-for-performance on 30-day mortality. The study used Medicare data and included patients from 252 hospitals that participated in the pay-for-performance program and 3,363 hospitals that did not participate in the program. In the simplest approach, one can determine 30-day mortality rates before and after the policy implementation for 252 hospitals, and compare those to see if mortality rate has improved or not. This pre-post design is susceptible to bias and results may not be solely attributed to the pay-for-performance policy.

In difference-in-difference analysis, patients from 3,363 hospitals serve as control groups. We can determine the surgical outcome rates before and after the policy change in two groups of hospitals: (i) a group of 252 hospitals where pay-for-performance policy has been implemented, and (ii) a group of 3,363 hospitals where pay-for-performance policy has not been implemented. The difference between the outcomes between two groups of hospitals [(T0-T1)-(C0-C1)] can be seen as the effect of policy implementation on improving outcomes. If there is no relationship between policy implementation and subsequent outcomes, then the difference-in-differences estimate is equal to zero. In contrast, if the policy is associated with improvement in outcomes, then the difference-in-difference estimator will be different from zero (Fig. 5.4). Finding an appropriate control group which has not been affected by the policy change can be a challenge when conducting difference-in-difference analysis.

Observational Research Study Examples

We provide two research study examples that used observational study design and different analytic methods to control for selection bias and confounding.

Study Example 1

Let's refer to study by Sheffield et al. [11]. The study investigated the association between intraoperative cholangiography (IOC) use during cholecystectomy and common duct injury. This retrospective cohort study used Medicare data. The exposure of interest (main independent variable) was IOC use and the outcome variable

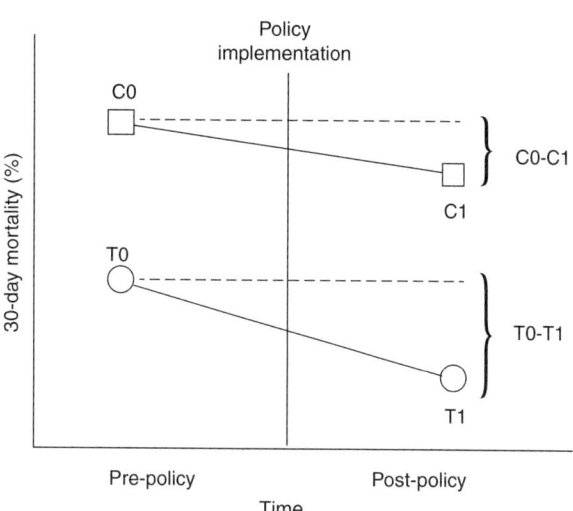

Fig. 5.4 Difference-in-difference analysis. *C0* Control group pre-policy, *C1* Control group post-policy, *T0* Treatment group pre-policy, *T1* Treatment group post-policy. Difference-in-difference estimator = (T0-T1) − (C0-C1). If the value of difference-in-difference estimator is zero, then the policy has no effect on reducing 30-day mortality. If value is greater than zero, it indicates the effectiveness of policy in reducing 30-day mortality

was common duct injury. The conceptual model for this study is depicted in Fig. 5.5. Previous studies using Medicare claims data had demonstrated an association between lack of IOC use and common duct injury. We hypothesized unmeasured confounders such as clinical indications for IOC (such as bilirubin levels and liver function tests) and factors that influence its use and successful completion (such as severe inflammation or aberrant anatomy) can explain the association between IOC use and common duct injury (see conceptual model, Fig. 5.5).

In the unadjusted model that did not control for any variables, patients with no IOC were 73 % (OR, 1.73; 95 % CI, 1.33–2.24) more likely to suffer a common duct injury compared to patients with IOC. Likewise, in the adjusted logistic regression model controlling for measured confounders, patients with no IOC were 76 % (OR, 1.76; 95 % CI, 1.34–2.32) more likely to suffer a common duct injury compared to patients with IOC. As is likely that patients operated in same hospitals may have similar outcome, we also used a 2-level model to control for clustering of patients within hospitals. However, this did not influence the magnitude or direction estimate of IOC use with common duct injury (Table 5.3). For regression models to control for confounding and selection bias, the predictors and confounders must be known and included in the model. In the above example, controlling for measured confounders did not significantly change the magnitude or direction of the odds ratio compared to those derived from the unadjusted model (Table 5.3, Fig. 5.5).

Instrumental variable analysis was used to control for potential unmeasured confounding including severity of disease, laboratory values, and other reasons that may have influenced IOC use. Authors hypothesized that use of IV analysis would attenuate the association between IOC and common duct injury. The percent of cholecystectomies performed with IOC at the hospital level was used as an IV. The percentage of hospital IOC use meets all three requirements for an IV. IOC use varied from 0 to 97 % across hospitals; as such, a patient's likelihood of receiving IOC was determined by the hospital level to which he or she presented

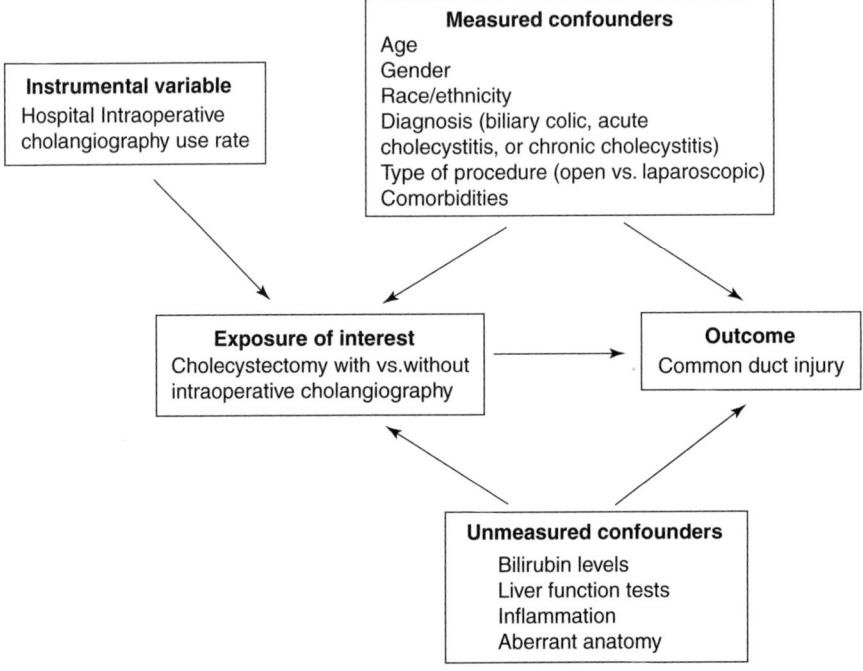

Fig. 5.5 Conceptual model for study evaluating association of intraoperative cholangiography (IOC) with common duct injury in Medicare beneficiaries. The exposure of interest is cholecystectomy with versus without IOC and the outcome is common duct injury. The measured and unmeasured confounders are shown in the figure. Hospital IOC use rate is an instrumental variable which only affects exposure of interest

Table 5.3 Association of exposure with outcome obtained using different analytic methods

	Intraoperative cholangiography and risk of common duct injury (Reference group: IOC use) (Sheffield et al. [11])	Endoscopic ultrasound and survival in pancreatic cancer (Reference group: No EUS use) (Parmar et al. [9])
Unadjusted model	1.73 (1.33–2.24)	0.67 (0.63–0.72)
Multivariable model	1.76 (1.34–2.32)	0.78 (0.73–0.84)
Multilevel model	1.79 (1.35–2.36)	Not done
Propensity score (PS)		
1:1 matching	Not done	0.77 (0.70–0.84)
PS regression adjustment	Not done	0.79 (0.74–0.85)
Instrumental variable	1.26 (0.81–1.96)	1.00 (0.73–1.36)

rather than the clinical characteristics. In the IV analysis, the association between IOC and common duct injury was significantly attenuated and no longer significant confirming our hypothesis of unmeasured confounding (OR, 1.26; 95 % CI,

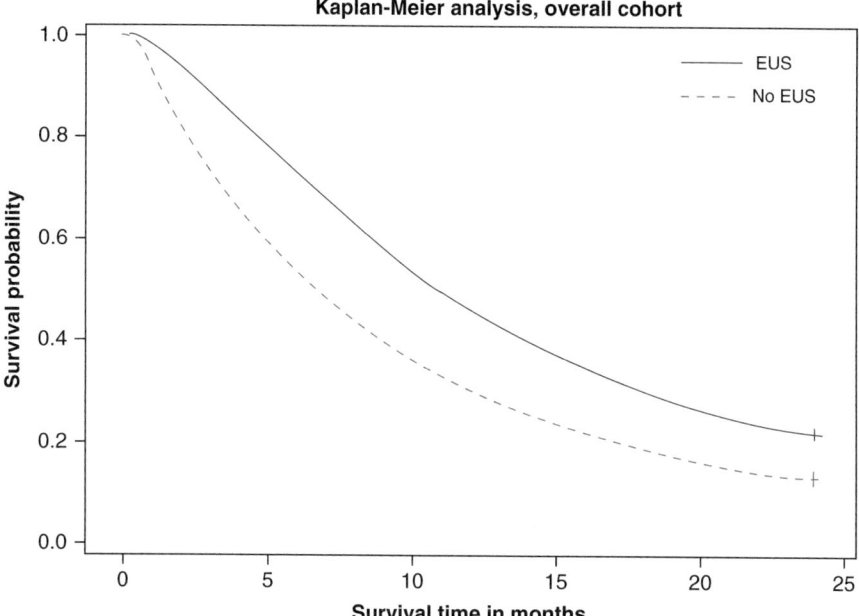

Fig. 5.6 Kaplan-Meier analysis of 2-year survival for patients with locoregional pancreatic adenocarcinoma, stratified by receipt of endoscopic ultrasound (EUS). The EUS group had improved survival (21.7% versus 12.8%, P<.0001)

0.81–1.96), in contrast to the results obtained from logistic regression and multilevel models (Table 5.3), which found an association between IOC and common duct injury.

Study Example 2

A study by Parmar et al. evaluated a previously reported association between receipt of endoscopic ultrasound (EUS) with survival in pancreatic cancer patients using SEER-Medicare data. The exposure of interest (main independent variable) was EUS and the outcome variable was time to death. It did not make clinical sense that receipt of a diagnostic test would influence survival, and the authors proposed unmeasured confounding.

In the unadjusted Kaplan-Meier survival analysis, the 2-year survival rate was higher in the EUS group (21.7% vs. 12.8%, p<0.0001, Fig. 5.6). The unadjusted hazard ratio for EUS was 0.67 (95% CI, 0.63–0.72), which means that EUS was associated with 33% improved survival in patients with pancreatic cancer compared to no EUS. When adjusting for the measured confounders, the association remained significant, but attenuated (Table 5.3).

To control for potential unmeasured confounding, the authors used propensity scores and instrumental variables to adjust for this potential confounding.

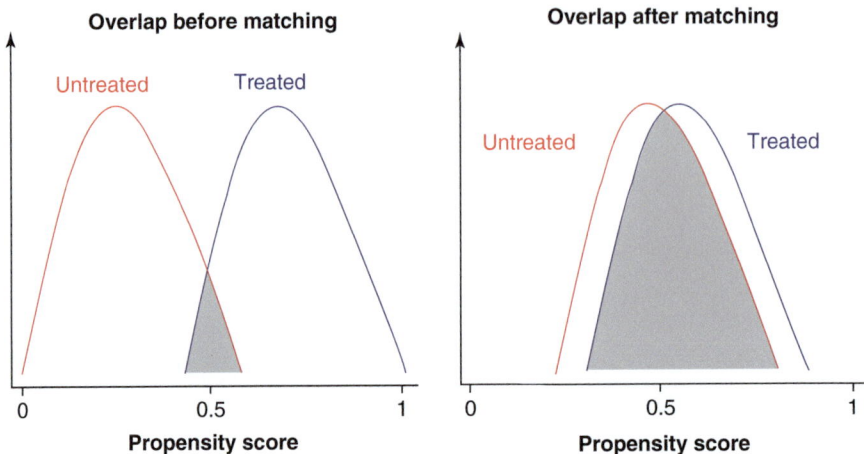

Fig. 5.7 Overlap of propensity score between endoscopic ultrasound (EUS) groups before and after matching. The overlap is low before matching and high after matching

In propensity score matching, 1,185 patients who received EUS were matched with 1,185 patients who did not receive EUS. This is 1:1 matching. Covariate balance across EUS and no EUS groups before and after propensity score matching was checked (Fig. 5.7). Both propensity score matching and propensity score regression adjustment had little influence on the hazard ratio. This is likely because propensity score does not control for unmeasured confounding. Percentage of EUS use at the health service area was used as an IV. In the IV analysis, the association between EUS with survival was no longer observed (HR, 1.00; 95 % CI, 0.73–1.36, Table 5.3).

Both examples showed that association between exposure and outcome was subject to unmeasured confounding. Traditional multivariable regression methods, multilevel models, and propensity score techniques did not control for unmeasured confounding. IV analysis removed unmeasured confounding to obtain unbiased treatment effect. It is important to know the strengths and limitations of the dataset, study design, and analytic technique while designing the study and interpreting the study results.

Summary

Understanding basic biostatistical methods is essential for both the research and clinical practice of a surgeon. Basic understanding of the methods discussed in this chapter will provide a basis for critically reading and reviewing the literature, designing studies, and performing simple and more advanced analysis in conjunction with a biostatistician.

Selected Reading

1. Afifi A, Clark VA, May S, editors. Computer-Aided Multivariate Analysis. 4th ed. Boca Raton: Chapman & Hall/CRC; 2004.
2. Agresti A, editor. An introduction to categorical data analysis. 2nd ed. Hoboken: Wiley; 2007.
3. Dawson B, Trapp RG, editors. Basic and clinical biostatistics. 4th ed. New York: McGraw Hill Companies Inc; 2004.
4. Dimick JB, Ryan AM. Methods for evaluating change in healthcare policy: the difference-in-difference approach. JAMA. 2014;312(22):2401–2.
5. Feinstein AR, Horwitz RI. A critique of the statistical evidence associating estrogens with endometrial cancer. Cancer Res. 1978;38(11 Pt 2):4001–5.
6. Giordano SH, Kuo Y, Duan Z, Hortobagyi G, Freeman J, Goodwin JS. Limits of observational data in determining outcomes from cancer therapy. Cancer. 2008;112:2456–66.
7. Jha AK, Joynt KE, Orav J, Epstein AM. The long term effect of premier pay for performance on patients outcomes. N Engl J Med. 2012;366(17):1606–15.
8. Kane RL. Understanding health care outcomes research. 2nd ed. Boston: Jones & Barlett Publishers, Inc.; 2006.
9. Parmar AD, Sheffield KM, Han Y, Vargas GM, Guturu PG, Kuo YF, Goodwin JS, Riall TS. Evaluating comparative effectiveness with observational data: endoscopic ultrasound and survival in pancreatic cancer. Cancer. 2013;119(21):3861–9.
10. Sheffield KM, Han Y, Kuo YF, Townsend Jr CM, Goodwin JS, Riall TS. Variation in the use of intraoperative cholangiography during cholecystectomy. J Am Coll Surg. 2012;214(4):668–79.
11. Sheffield KM, Riall TS, Han Y, Kuo YF, Townsend Jr CM, Goodwin JS. Association between cholecystectomy with vs without intraoperative cholangiography and risk of common duct injury. JAMA. 2013;310(8):812–20.
12. Strom BL, Kimmel SE, Hennessy S. Pharmacoepidemiology. 5th ed. Wiley-Blackwell. Oxford, UK; 2012.

Chapter 6
Animal Models for Surgical Research

Andrea A. Hayes-Jordan

Murine

Transgenic Models

The quintessential animal model for transgenic mice is the rip-tag model developed by Douglas Hanahan. This model was developed in the 1980s [1] and continues, after almost 40 years to sustain his research including hundreds of manuscripts published in peer review journals, continuous NIH funding for four decades, and many articles in Cell, Nature and Science. Transgenic mice carrying oncogenes that reproducibly elicit tumors of specific cell types has provided a new format for studying multi-step tumorigenesis. In one of these models, transgenic mice expressing an oncogene in the cells of the pancreatic islets heritably recapitulate a progression from normality to hyperplasia to neoplasia. Angiogenic activity first appears in a subset of hyperplastic islets before the onset of tumor formation. A few hyperplastic islets become angiogenic in vitro at a time when such islets are neovascularized in vivo and at a frequency that correlates closely with subsequent tumor incidence. This supports the concept that induction of angiogenesis is an important step in carcinogenesis.

What is a transgene? And what is a transgenic mouse?

A transgene is an exogenous gene delivered into the genome of another organism. An exogenous gene is injected directly into an embryo or cells at early embryonic stage using a microscopic needle. In this particular model, the gene used is an insulin gene in order to directly target the beta cells of the islet of Langerhans of the pancreas and as such that is where the tumors will develop. Simian Virus 40 (SV40) is a known oncogene, meaning it transforms any cell to which is introduced into a

---

A.A. Hayes-Jordan, MD
Professor of Surgery and Pediatrics, Department of Surgical Oncology, UT MD Anderson Cancer Center, 1400 Pressler St, Unit 1484, Houston, TX 77030, USA
e-mail: ahjordan@mdanderson.org

cancer cell. In this strain the rat insulin promoter (RIP) directs expression of the SV40 Large T antigen transgene (TAg) to beta cells of the pancreatic islets. Following the transfer into fertilized mouse eggs of recombinant genes composed of the upstream region of the rat insulin II gene linked to sequences coding for the large-T antigen of SV40, large-T antigen is detected exclusively in the beta cells of the endocrine pancreas of transgenic mice. The SV40 TAg oncogene is expressed beginning at ~ E8 (mice at embryo day 8 of gestation). The mice are systemically tolerant to large T antigen. The alpha and beta cells normally found in the islets of Langerhans are rare and disordered. Well-vascularized beta cell tumors arise in mice harboring and inheriting these hybrid oncogenes. Hyperplastic islets begin to appear by 3–4 weeks of age. Angiogenic islets (Islet cells that are forming new blood vessels) (8–12% of the total) arise from hyperplastic/dysplastic islets by switching on angiogenesis. Solid tumors (~3% of the islets) emerge at about 10 weeks as small, encapsulated adenomas that progress into large adenomas by 12–13 weeks of age in postnatal rats. Development to vascularized invasive carcinomas occurs less frequently. This model has many virtues as a prototype for testing experimental therapeutics, although it will not necessarily be suitable for all drugs, such as oncogene-specific inhibitors. The advantages of the model are its 14-week time course, the 100% penetrance of invasive cancer, and the synchronous appearance of dysplasias, angiogenic switching, adenomas, and carcinomas. The multifocality of the target tissue (the 400 islets) and the lesions that develop allow quantification of tumor development. Other non-cancer genes can be used as the transgene to target expression in particular tissue types.

Xenograft Models

Xenograft animal models are models in which, human cells, or cells from another species is injected into, usually, an immunocompromised animal that will prevent rejection of the cells or tissue. These models come in two versions, heterotopic and orthotopic. In heterotopic models, for convenience and ease of observation, human cells grown in culture or morselated human tissue, is injected subdermally or subcutaneously in a mouse or rat lacking T-cells, B-Cells, Natural Killer (NK) cells, a thymus, or any or all of the above.

Subcutaneous implantation allows visible growth and the addition of treatment, at any time desired by the investigator so the desired result can be measured without sacrificing the mice until the end of the experiment. The disadvantage of this model is that it does not completely recapitulate the human clinical condition. Although many heterotopic models are described, if you are to convince your reviewers for example that your treatment in mice will be effective in human trials, the model must be convincingly similar to the human condition. The use of heterotopic models is usually utilized as additional preliminary data to verify compelling in vitro findings. If one takes liver cells for example, and injects them under the skin, one cannot expect that it will be subject to the same micro-environmental stressors that occur in

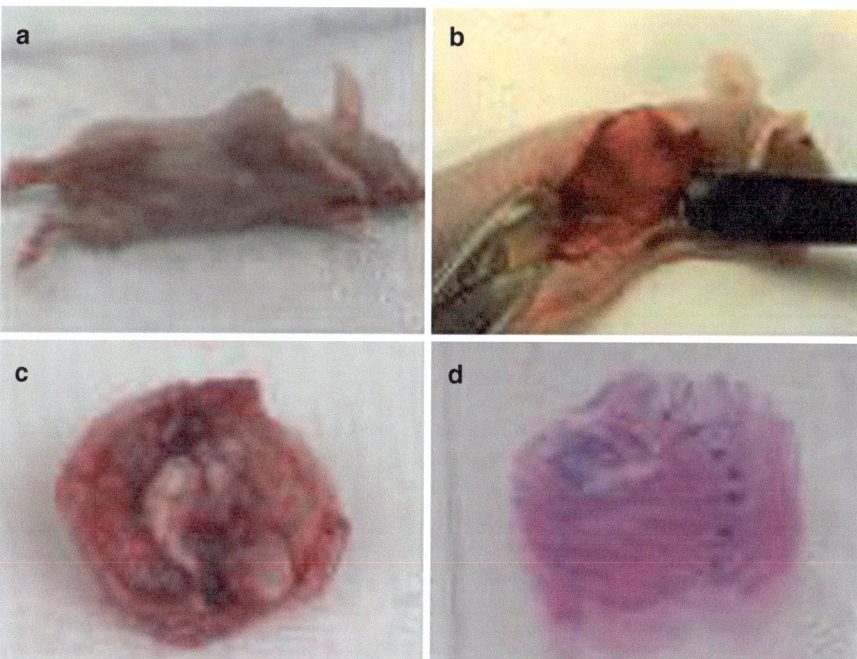

Fig. 6.1 (**a**) A nude mouse 3 weeks after injection of 500,000 human Ewing's sarcoma cells into the rib. (**b**) The tumor is exposed after skin is cut, verifying the orthotopic position. (**c**) The thoracic cavity has been isolated with the heart removed arrows identify bilateral pulmonary metastasis. (**d**) *Arrow* show small blue cell tumor among ribs imbedded in muscle and bone of the chest wall [2]

the liver. Liver cells should be injected into liver, colon cells into the colon, etc. Thus orthotopic xenograft models more closely mimic human presentation. Cells from bone tumors or liver tumors are injected into the bone or liver respectively (Fig. 6.1). This allows one to study the growth and differentiation of ones cell of interest, in its own native microenvironment. This has been shown to be much more accurate and clinically relevant than heterotopic models [3].

If intracavitary organs are being studied, to avoid having to sacrifice the animal or perform survival surgery to evaluate the results of one's treatment, non-invasive imaging can be used. Cells of interest are transfected with a color 'tag' for which there are many to choose. One of the most popular is luciferase. Luciferase or green fluorescent protein (GFP) is inserted in a vector which can be then used for transfection into mammalian cells. Luciferase is the enzyme for the substrate luciferin. When the animal is injected with luciferin, a signal is emitted from the cells which have been transfected with luciferase which can then be photographed in the appropriate imager. The signal intensity of the light emitted can then be quantified [2] (Fig. 6.2).

Recently, orthotopic xenograft models have become the standard in oncologic research. One of the best examples is a metastatic colon cancer model established by colorectal surgeons at the Cleveland Clinic. This model was established in 1996,

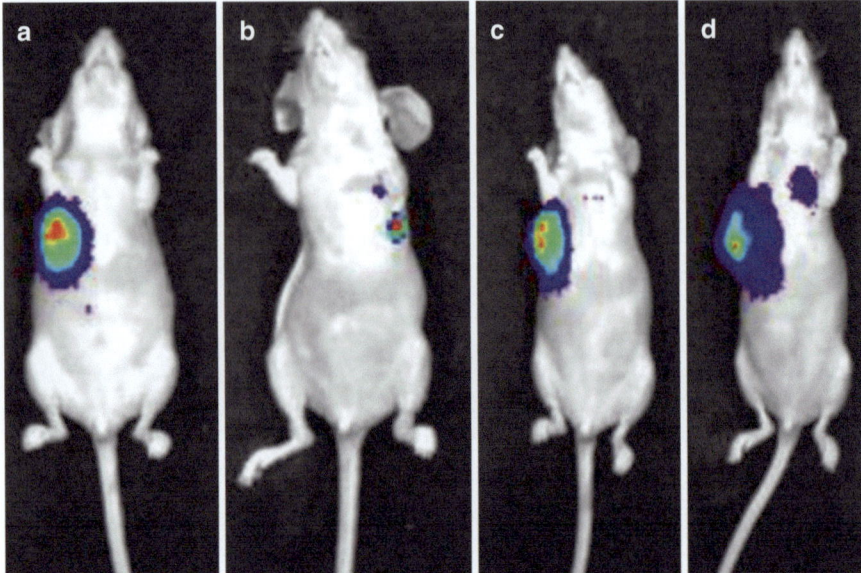

Fig. 6.2 Luciferase vector transfected TC-71 Ewing's sarcoma cells injected into the rib of nude mice (**a**) *Filled arrow* indicates chest wall tumor 20 days after orthotopic injection of TC-71 Ewing's sarcoma cells into the rib. No pulmonary metastases are seen (65 % of mice have this phenotype) (**b**) *Line arrow* indicates early pulmonary metastasis at 18 days after injection of TC-71 Ewing's sarcoma cells. No chest wall tumor is seen (25–30 % of mice have this phenotype) (**c, d**). Chest wall tumor and pulmonary metastasis at 16 and 22 days post injection (less than 10 % of mice have this phenotype). cells were transfected with luciferase, then injected into the rib of nude mice. Mice were injected with luciferin prior to imaging. The intensity of bioluminescent color correlates with tumor size

and subsequently improved upon by a Korean colorectal surgery group in 2012 [4, 5]. Syngeneic rats were injected intra-splenically, with poorly differentiated colon adenocarcinoma cells. In 4–12 weeks, liver metastases were seen in all lobes of the liver. The choice of using the splenic vein was to easily access the portal venous system, which is a known delivery conduit for metastatic cells from the colon. Dr Kim modified this approach by injecting the colon carcinoma cells directly into the portal vein using a 30 gauge needle. This again reproducibly yielded multiple liver metastases (Fig. 6.3).

This modification and improvement in an animal model, highlights the need to modify your research approach as necessary to achieve more accuracy.

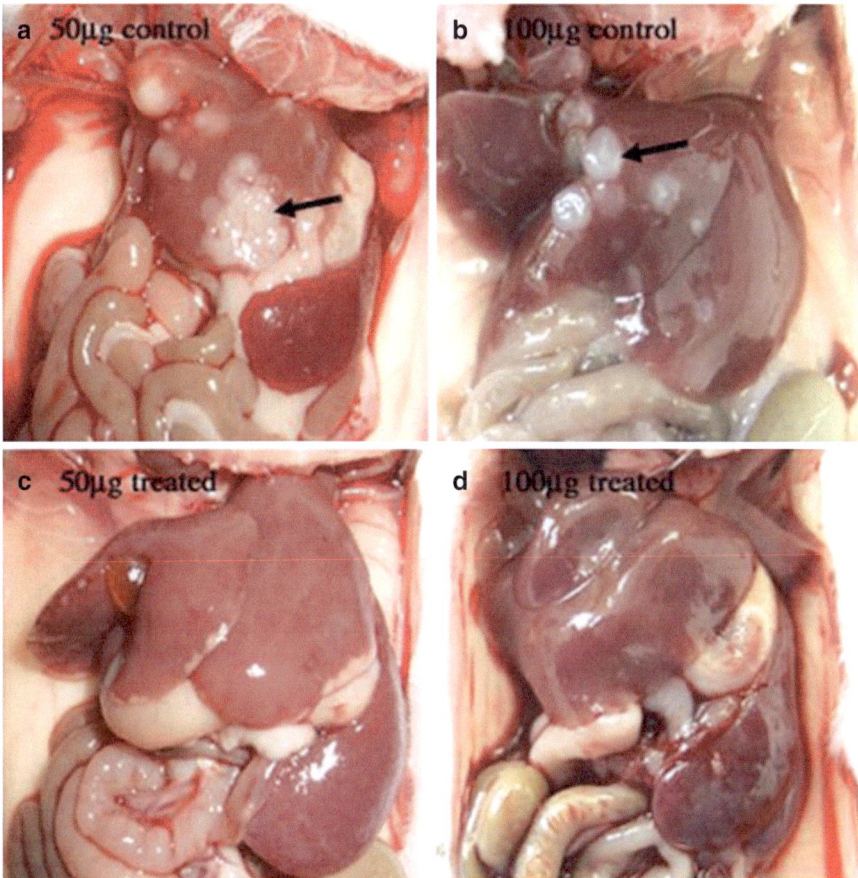

Fig. 6.3 Representative photos of livers from the mice treated with 50 and 100 µg of CpG (**c, d**) and from their corresponding control groups (**a, b**). Note that hepatic metastasized tumor nodules were clustered and easily visualized on the liver surface, but were either significantly less or absent in mice treated with CpG (obtained from Elsevier with permission)

Non-cancer Models

Larger animal models are often used to perform new minimally invasive surgical techniques or assess the safety of new implants or devices. Pigs are very useful for these types of studies. For example, pigs can be used to study minimally invasive techniques or use of new allograft replacement materials for ventral hernias. Adult sheep or pigs are large enough to mimic abdominal or thoracic surgery [6] of humans, and techniques established in these models are easily transferable to humans. Piglets are close to the size of infants or children and are used for some pediatric studies. Fetal and neonatal piglet skin is also useful for wound healing assays since fetal skin exhibits scarless wound healing.

There are a few disadvantages of large animal models. First, the presence of a veterinary team to be present before, during and after the operations to care for the well-being of the animal is necessary. This limits the number of cases one can do in 1 day to one or two, compared to murine studies where up to ten times the number of animal assays can be completed in 1 day and recovery of mice or rats undergoing a general anesthetic can be done by the investigator. Also, cost is significantly more. Mice can cost $10–$15 per animal including feeding, and larger animals such as pigs, sheep or dogs, cost $500–$5000 each.

Animal models are also useful for studying the physiologic response to injury. One example is a model developed and utilized by trauma surgeons to study closed head injury. Dr Cox and his team have been able to study the brain after closed head injury [7, 8]. A special device used for controlled closed injury to the unilateral cranium of C57/Bl6 mice is administered. The mice are then subject to partial craniectomy (as is performed by neurosurgeons in some closed head injuries) followed by various treatment strategies to repair the damaged microglia using autologous mesenchymal stem cells and other therapies. This model has allowed detailed study of the microglia/macrophage interaction as well as microscopic studies of the effect on the blood–brain barrier. The data from these successful experiments led to human clinical trials in pediatric trauma, using stem cell therapy to repair the brain after brain injury from trauma.

Clinical Physiology and Phenotypic Mimicry Models

If there is a known clinical 'trigger' for the disease entity you wish to study, one can exaggerate this 'trigger' in an animal model. Recapitulating this in a murine model is done and the similar phenotypic outcome that is seen in clinical scenarios in humans is documented. For example, hypoxia and formula feeds are known to be risk factors for necrotizing enterocolitis (NEC) and thus these conditions can be reproduced in the rat and causing the same appearance and physiology of NEC in the intestines of the rat [9, 10].

Another example is gram negative bacterial overload causing sepsis. Animals are infused the known endotoxin that is expanded by gram negative bacteria, and whichever novel treatment one is evaluating can be delivered and studied in this model. Cardiac, pulmonary or intestinal end organ effects can be measured. Another model of polymicrobial sepsis is cecal puncture in a mouse; this model can mimic severe sepsis [11, 12]. These animals acutely deteriorate after the cecum is ligated and punctured. Then, the systemic inflammation can be measured by tumor necrosis factor, interleukin-6, interleukin-10, as well as other inflammatory cytokines. In this model however, the initial mortality of the animals, which can be up to half, is limiting. Here again is another technique that has been modified. Dr Liu discovered that instead of using a regular hypodermic needle, if one uses a three sided needle, many fewer animals die immediately, that therefore allows for more efficient investigation in this particular model [12].

Other models include those in which mechanical occlusion of vasculature and blood flow or hollow viscus, as a survival surgery, then mimics perfusion related or developmental related structural abnormalities. This includes ischemia reperfusion and intestinal developmental models. A high level of technical skill is required for these models therefore these are well suited to be executed by a surgical investigator. In rat or mice models almost no blood loss is tolerated for survival surgery to be successful. Physiological changes can be measured at various times after temporary or permanent occlusion of vasculature and the results of drug interventions measured.

Alternative Vertebrate Models

Zebrafish have become a popular and excellent model to study development, cancer and genetics. The zebrafish has become prized because its transparent embryo develops outside the mother's body. This transparency allows minute to minute visualization of the cardiovascular, including blood flow, and structural changes that occur in 'real time'. Because the zebrafish is a vertebrate animal, it has become a valuable resource for identifying genes involved in human disease.

Thomas Bartman and colleagues use the powerful tools afforded by zebrafish genetics to examine the early steps of heart valve formation. In the process, they provide evidence for a causal relationship between the early function of the heart and its final structure. Using a fluorescent molecular marker highly expressed in the developing heart, the authors found mutations that result in valve defects, and identified a fish mutant they named cardiofunk (cfk). Genetic mapping of cfk showed that the abnormality was caused by a mutation in a gene encoding a novel actin molecule that is most closely related to the actins found in muscle cells. Actin is involved in muscle contraction; so these results suggest that muscle contraction in the embryonic heart is intimately involved in heart development. Valve or septal defects represent 40% of cardiac anomalies in humans. By studying zebrafish, Bartman and colleagues suggest some of these defects may result from congenital defects affecting very early heart function [13].

Zebrafish are being used to study in cancer by Nancy Hopkins of the Massachusetts Institute of Technology. Her group has created over 500 lines of zebrafish with lesions in key genes involved in development and used them to identify a group of genes that predispose the fish to cancer. Using close observation while cultivating some of these mutant lines, this team noticed that an abnormally large percentage of

Fig. 6.4 Nearly transparent zebrafish

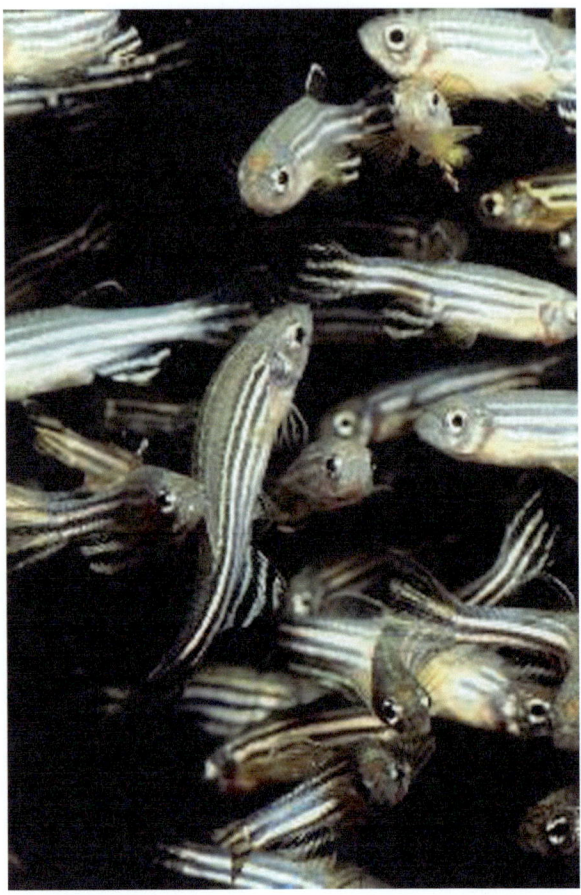

fish died young, whereas the surviving fish in these lines developed large, highly invasive malignant tumors. This facilitated the discovery of a ribosomal gene (rp) essential for embryonic development. Given the high degree of conservation of genes and pathways among vertebrates, it is possible that rp mutations also raise cancer risk in humans. Together, these results demonstrate that the tiny freshwater workhorse of developmental biology has a promising future as a model system for human cancer (Fig. 6.4) [13].

References

1. Hanahan D. Dissecting multistep tumorigenesis in transgenic mice. Annu Rev Genet. 1988;22:479–519.

2. Wang YX, Mandal D, Wang S, Hughes D, Pollock RE, Lev D, et al. Inhibiting platelet-derived growth factor beta reduces Ewing's sarcoma growth and metastasis in a novel orthotopic human xenograft model. In Vivo. 2009;23(6):903–9.
3. Fidler IJ. Seed and soil revisited: contribution of the organ microenvironment to cancer metastasis. Surg Oncol Clin N Am. 2001;10(2):257–69, vii–viiii.
4. Brand MI, Casillas S, Dietz DW, Milsom JW, Vladisavljevic A. Development of a reliable colorectal cancer liver metastasis model. J Surg Res. 1996;63(2):425–32.
5. Kim IY, Yan X, Tohme S, Ahmed A, Cordon-Cardo C, Shantha Kumara HM, et al. CpG ODN, Toll like receptor (TLR)-9 agonist, inhibits metastatic colon adenocarcinoma in a murine hepatic tumor model. J Surg Res. 2012;174(2):284–90.
6. Feretis C, Kalantzopoulos D, Koulouris P, Chandakas S, Sideris M, Papalois A. Experimenal studies of peroral transgastric abdominal. Anna Gastroenterol. 2006;1(19):60–5.
7. Walker PA, Bedi SS, Shah SK, Jimenez F, Xue H, Hamilton JA, Smith P, Thomas CP, Mays RW, Pati S, Cox Jr CS. Intravenous multipotent adult progenitor cell therapy after traumatic brain injury: modulation of the resident microglia population. J Neuroinflammation. 2012;9:228.
8. Fischer UM, Harting MT, Jimenez F, et al. Pulmonary passage is a major obstacle for intravenous stem cell delivery: the pulmonary first pass effect. Stem Cells Dev. 2009;18(5):683–92.
9. Lim JC, Golden JM, Ford HR. Pathogenesis of neonatal necrotizing enterocolitis. Pediatr Surg Int. 2015;31(6):509–18.
10. Lugo B, Ford HR, Grishin A. Molecular signaling in necrotizing enterocolitis: regulation of intestinal COX-2 expression. J Pediatr Surg. 2007;42(7):1165–71.
11. Lewis AJ, Yuan D, Zhang X, Angus DC, Rosengart MR, Seymour CW. Use of biotelemetry to define physiology-based deterioration thresholds in a murine cecal ligation and puncture model of sepsis. Critical Care Med. 2016;44(6):e420–31.
12. Liu X, Wang N, Wei G, Fan S, Lu Y, Zhu Y, et al. Consistency and pathophysiological characterization of a rat polymicrobial sepsis model via the improved cecal ligation and puncture surgery. Int Immunopharmacol. 2016;32:66–75.
13. Bartman T, Walsh EC, Wen KK, McKane M, Ren J, Alexander J, et al. Early myocardial function affects endocardial cushion development in zebrafish. PLoS Biol. 2004;2(5):E129.

Chapter 7
Health Services Research

Caprice C. Greenberg and Justin B. Dimick

Introduction

Health services research (HSR) is defined by the Institute of Medicine as a multidisciplinary field of inquiry, both basic and applied, that examines the use, costs, quality, accessibility, delivery, organization, financing, and outcomes of health care services to increase knowledge and understanding of the structure, processes, and outcomes of health services for individuals and populations. As suggested by this definition, surgeon-scientists may have a strategic advantage in health services & outcomes research because of our nuanced understanding of the clinical context, including diseases and the delivery system. As a result, our experience is that surgeon-scientists can build on this advantage to compete successfully for external grant funding in this discipline.

In this chapter, we will provide an overview of the field of HSR in surgery, often also termed surgical outcomes research. While "HSR" and "outcomes research" mean different things to different people, they are often used interchangeably, and we will do so in this chapter. To ground our discussion, we suggest a conceptual model that identifies three core components of the U.S. healthcare system: (1) disease management; (2) the local micro-system in which treatment is provided; and (3) the policy environment (i.e., macro-system) in which healthcare is delivered. Combinations of these three components can be used to define the major scientific

---

C.C. Greenberg, M.D., MPH (✉)
Wisconsin Surgical Outcomes Research (WiSOR) Program, Department of Surgery,
University of Wisconsin Hospitals & Clinics, 600 Highland Avenue, Clinical Science Center,
K6/100, Madison, WI 53792-1690, USA

J.B. Dimick, M.D., MPH
Center for Healthcare Outcomes and Policy, and the Department of Surgery,
University of Michigan, Ann Arbor, MI, USA

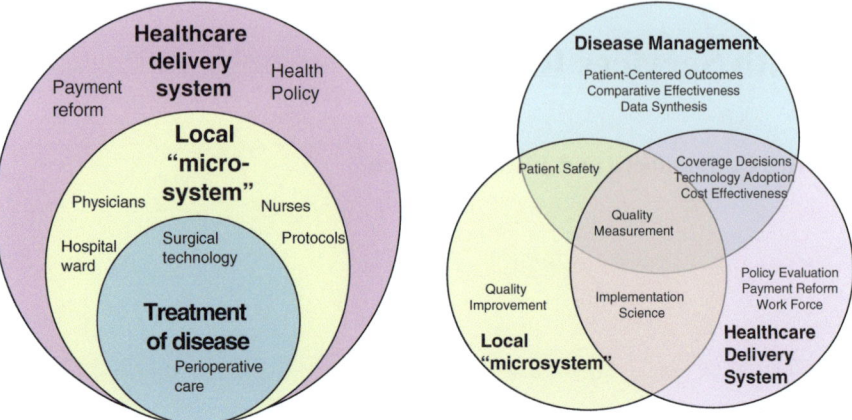

Fig. 7.1 Conceptual model for the discipline of Health Services Research (HSR). Panel (**a**) depicts how the key elements of our healthcare system interact: (1) disease management; (2) the local micro-system in which treatments are provided; and (3) the policy environment (i.e., macro-system) in which health care is delivered. These same three elements form the basic domains of the discipline of HSR which is dedicated to understanding the system and approach to care provided at the individual patient, local, and healthcare delivery system levels. Panel (**b**) depicts the variety of intellectual disciplines that are considered health services research and how each relates to one of the three elements of the healthcare system or their intersection

Table 7.1 The domains and intellectual disciplines that comprise health services research

Domain	Intellectual discipline	Areas of focus
Evaluating disease management (Patient-level)	Comparative effectiveness research	Pragmatic clinical trials
		Cluster randomized trials
		Observational studies
	Patient-centered outcomes	Quality of life
		Patient satisfaction
		Shared decision-making
	Data synthesis	Meta-analysis
		Decision analysis
Understanding local provision of care (Micro-system)	Quality measurement	Public reporting
		Benchmarking outcomes
	Implementation science	
	Patient safety	Systems Engineering
		Human Factors
		System Redesign
Healthcare delivery system (Macro-system)	Policy evaluation	Payment reform
		Coverage decisions
	Work force	Forecasting future needs
		Regional variations

Table 7.2 Summary of research techniques used in surgical health services research

Quantitative	Qualitative
Clinical trial design	Focus groups
Meta-analysis	Key informant interviews
Decision analysis	Field observations
Cost-effectiveness analysis	Grounded theory analysis
Survey/questionnaire administration	Modified Delphi technique
Large database analyses	
Advanced statistical modeling	
Econometrics	

HSR uses a variety of both quantitative and qualitative techniques. This table provides an example of basic techniques utilized throughout the three major domains of HSR

domains of HSR (Fig. 7.1). For each of the three major domains, we will provide a brief overview and discuss the intellectual disciplines and research tools necessary to conduct high-level studies in that area (Tables 7.1 and 7.2).

Patient-Level Questions: Evaluating Disease Management

Overview

One domain of health services research evaluates the treatment of disease, but does so at a population-level under "real-world" conditions or from the patient's point of view. HSR often provides important data that cannot be generated from traditional clinical trials. Traditional randomized clinical trials are "efficacy" trials designed to evaluate a given treatment approach under the best case scenario and thus adhere to strict inclusion and exclusion criteria. "Effectiveness" trials are equally important and evaluate how well a given treatment approach works outside of a controlled trial when all patients are considered. This area of HSR is primarily referred to as comparative effectiveness research (CER) and its closely aligned partner patient-centered outcomes research (PCOR). Another important area of inquiry is data synthesis, including such techniques as meta-analyses and decision analyses, which aim to answer questions by combining data generated from multiple studies in a scientifically rigorous way.

Intellectual Disciplines and Research Tools

Comparative Effectiveness Research

The Federal Coordinating Council for Comparative Effectiveness Research defines comparative effectiveness research (CER) as the conduct and synthesis of research comparing the benefits and harms of different interventions and strategies to prevent, diagnose, treat and monitor health conditions in 'real world' settings [1]. This type of research seeks to understand which treatment approach is the most beneficial to patients outside of clinical trials. CER must compare at least two different approaches to determine which has the potential to be the optimal choice. CER can be either retrospective or prospective and can evaluate any type of intervention including drugs, operations, or even approaches to healthcare delivery.

Retrospective CER primarily uses large population-based datasets, including patient registries, administrative data, or health insurance claims data to evaluate outcomes based on several different approaches to care when there is equipoise in current clinical practice. For example, a 2009 study published in *Journal of the American Medical Association* compared the effectiveness of open versus minimally invasive prostatectomy [2]. The treatment of prostate cancer tops most lists of the most critical questions to address in CER given the similar outcomes observed with very divergent approaches to care including radiation, surgery, and clinical observation. By combining the disease-specific variables in the Surveillance Epidemiology and End Results (SEER) registry data with longitudinal Medicare claims data, the authors were able to compare both short and long-term outcomes following each surgical approach. Open prostatectomy was associated with longer length of stay, higher rates of in-hospital complications, and higher rates of stricture, but lower rates of incontinence and erectile dysfunction. Importantly, between 2003 and 2007, the rate of minimally invasive surgery for prostatectomy increased from 9 to 43 % emphasizing the importance of a timely evaluation of this new surgical technique. The rapid adoption of minimally invasive prostatectomy occurred before a randomized clinical trial could have been performed and its remarkable utilization rate precludes the performance of such a trial at this point. CER offers an important approach to providing much needed data on new surgical techniques as illustrated by this example.

The major challenge in retrospective CER is accounting for observed and unobserved confounding variables. In traditional clinical trials, imbalances in baseline characteristics between the different treatment arms are minimized by randomization. In CER, investigators use a variety of tools to adjust for confounders (or characteristics that may differ between the two groups of patients and lead to observed differences in outcome) and approximate randomization as closely as possible. Examples of such techniques include multivariable models, propensity scores, and instrumental variables.

Prospective CER can be randomized or non-randomized, such as a prospective observational cohort study. Randomized CER is also often called "pragmatic clinical trials", to reflect the fact that they are conducted under "real world" conditions and practice. Inclusion and exclusion criteria are minimal if they exist at all. Randomization may take place at any level – meaning patients may be randomized to one treatment or another individually or randomization may take place at the level of the physician, clinic, or institution. This later type of randomization is referred to as a "cluster randomized" trial and represents an important approach in CER and other types of prospective randomized research.

Patient-Centered Outcomes Research

The importance of the patient perspective and experience in our evaluation of surgical and other health outcomes has been expanding rapidly over the last few years. With the creation of the Patient Centered Outcomes Research Institute (PCORI) in the Affordable Care Act in March 2010, PCOR has rapidly gained wide spread attention. It has really redefined our approach to scientific inquiry by requiring partnerships between patients and other stakeholders and the investigative team. According to PCORI, Patient-Centered Outcomes Research (PCOR) helps people and their caregivers communicate and make informed healthcare decisions, allowing their voices to be heard in assessing the value of healthcare options. This research answers patient-centered questions, such as [3]:

1. "Given my personal characteristics, conditions, and preferences, what should I expect will happen to me?"
2. "What are my options, and what are the potential benefits and harms of those options?"
3. "What can I do to improve the outcomes that are most important to me?"
4. "How can clinicians and the care delivery systems they work in help me make the best decisions about my health and health care?"

To answer these questions, PCOR:

- Assesses the benefits and harms of preventive, diagnostic, therapeutic, palliative, or health delivery system interventions to inform decision making, highlighting comparisons and outcomes that matter to people;
- Is inclusive of an individual's preferences, autonomy, and needs, focusing on outcomes that people notice and care about such as survival, function, symptoms, and health-related quality of life;
- Incorporates a wide variety of settings and diversity of participants to address individual differences and barriers to implementation and dissemination; and
- Investigates (or may investigate) optimizing outcomes while addressing burden to individuals, availability of services, technology, and personnel, and other stakeholder perspectives.

This is an extremely comprehensive definition that can be difficult to practically apply. As a result, it may be simpler to paraphrase PCORI by considering PCOR to be "research that addresses the questions and concerns most relevant to patients and involves patients, caregivers, clinicians, and other healthcare stakeholders, along with researchers, throughout the process". At least 10 % of the current 508 research projects funded by PCORI are either investigating a surgical issue or held by a surgical principal investigator [3]. Surgical research is closer to 1 % of the NIH budget, again suggesting PCOR and other types of HSR are a natural fit for surgery.

There are several aspects of surgery that make it particularly well-suited for CER and PCOR. First, we have a discrete, single intervention (operation) that can be identified using billing and administrative data including a date of service. Consider for example the ease with which one can identify an operation compared to a change in anti-hypertensive medication. Additionally, surgical outcomes tend to be important over a shorter period of time, even in-hospital endpoints are meaningful for surgeons, and again more easily identified and more easily directly linked to the intervention.

Data Synthesis

One of the goals of health services research is to provide the data and information required to make decisions that are faced in the everyday care of patients. As such, another domain of HSR is dedicated to synthesizing data that is generated in other settings to answer a particular question – often one that cannot be answered by a clinical trial. Meta-analyses provide a systematic, rigorous way to combine the results from a number of independent studies to estimate the overall effect of a particular treatment. By using statistical methodologies to combine the results of a number of smaller studies, power can be increased such that Type 2 error is minimized and an effect may be observed.

Decision analysis is another important area of HSR that was adopted from economics and uses data from previously published studies to try to answer questions that cannot be answered using traditional clinical trials. There are a number of different models that can be employed in a decision analysis including decision trees or state transition models (the most commonly used one being Markov models). Decision analyses provide a mechanism for determining what approach will maximize value. A number of branch points, either decisions (e.g., surgery or chemotherapy) or chance (e.g., post-operative complication or no post-operative complication) are encountered along the course and previously published estimates or other sources are used to provide values or likelihoods for each option at a decision point.

The "Micro-system": Understanding and Optimizing the Local Provision of Care

Overview

In the previous section, we discussed the evaluation of the impact of different treatments on patient disease. Although such research is important for deciding which treatments are best for patients, there is a growing body of research suggesting a large gap between what is known to be the best and what is done in actual practice. There are numerous studies documenting that the quality of care provided varies widely across populations within the U.S. healthcare system. Populations can be defined by patient characteristics such as race or socioeconomic status or by where care is provided – the institution or even the region of the country. Thus, whether patients receive high quality care, consistent with best medical knowledge, is often a function of the local healthcare system.

This second domain we will consider, the local system of care, is comprised of the providers, resources, and systems that collectively provide care. There are several attributes of providers and processes that increase (or decrease) the likelihood that patients will receive appropriate care. We consider systems "high quality" if they are aligned to promote adherence to best practices and thereby achieve the best outcomes. Much of the research in this area has traditionally been descriptive – what might be considered patterns of care research – depicting racial disparities or documenting the relationship between hospital volume and outcome – or focused on defining ways to measure quality. As our understanding of variations in care and ability to quantify quality has become more sophisticated, we have recently moved into a more interventional approach to this type of work, focusing on disciplines such as quality improvement and implementation science.

Intellectual Disciplines and Research Tools

Disparities

A large body of research shows that certain racial and ethnic groups have worse surgical outcomes compared to others. Although for some diseases, differences in outcomes can be explained in small part by differences in biology, a much larger component of the disparities problem in the US is due to the healthcare system, both the micro- and the macro-systems in which care is delivered. The importance of investigating and intervening at both a local and national level is illustrated by the depiction (Fig. 7.1) of this discipline at the intersection of the local micro- and macro-system level.

Disparities in access and quality of care exist within institutions and there is growing evidence to support complicated social and cultural etiologies. For example, using data from the National Initiative for Cancer Care Quality, we found that disparities in rates of reconstruction following mastectomy for breast cancer based on age, race, and education were related to the likelihood that providers discussed reconstruction with their patients [4]. Once the discussions takes place, lower rates of reconstruction were observed in older and Hispanic patients and those who were born outside of the United States suggesting other factors at play, such as a cultural preference or language barriers. Issues such as trust and communication have been demonstrated to vary according to race and play a role in the patient-provider interactions in a number of diseases.

Additionally, a growing body of research suggests that our healthcare delivery system remains segregated, with referral patterns directing blacks and Hispanics to lower quality hospitals. The following example provides clear evidence of these segregated referral patterns. Liu and colleagues used the California hospital discharge database to investigate access to high volume hospitals (as a proxy for quality). In this study published in the *Journal of the American Medical Association*, blacks were significantly less likely than whites to receive care at high-volume hospitals for six of the ten operations (relative risk [RR] range, 0.40–0.72), while Hispanics were significantly less likely to receive care at high-volume hospitals for nine of ten operations (RR range, 0.46–0.88) [5]. In subsequent studies, this general finding of less access to high quality providers among blacks & Hispanics vs. whites has been proven true for a broad array of surgical (and medical) conditions. Such entrenched referral patterns are an important, but often overlooked, attribute of our healthcare delivery system.

Quality Measurement

Given the substantial importance of quality measurement to hospital administrators and policymakers, it is no surprise that many surgical investigators focus on this field. Surgeons have learned that understanding how best to measure our own performance gives us a "seat at the table" that we would not have otherwise. Thus, surgical performance assessment remains an important area of scientific focus.

Most often, surgical quality is measured according to the Donabedian triad of structure, process, and outcome. Structure refers to fixed attributes of the system (e.g., hospital volume, surgeon specialty). Process refers to the details of care associated with good outcomes (e.g., adherence to recommended perioperative antibiotics). Outcomes represent the end results of care, most often morbidity and mortality, but they can also include functional status, quality of life, and patient satisfaction.

The most widely cited example of research linking hospital structure and outcome is by Birkmeyer et al. in a paper published in the *New England Journal of Medicine* in 2002 [6]. He used national Medicare claims data to study the relationship between hospital volume and risk-adjusted mortality for 14 high-risk surgical conditions. Although there were many prior studies demonstrating the volume-outcome relationship, this paper was the first to examine a broad range of procedures in a systematic way. Perhaps the greatest contribution of this study was the finding that the strength of the volume-mortality relationship varied across procedures. For some rare procedures, such as pancreatectomy and esophagectomy, the relationship was quite strong, with greater than 10 % mortality differences between high and low volume hospitals. In contrast, for coronary artery bypass surgery and carotid endarterectomy, the differences were only approximately 1 % between high and low volume hospitals.

Much of the research on processes of care in surgery focuses on identifying which "matter" in terms of optimizing outcomes. For example, a high profile JAMA study by Stulberg et al., evaluated the impact of the Surgical Care Improvement Program (SCIP) measures on risk-adjusted outcomes [7]. Stulberg and colleagues used an inpatient administrative database from Premier, Inc., to study the relationship between SCIP processes (e.g., appropriate selection, timing, and redosing of prophylactic antibiotics) and postoperative wound infections. They found that none of the individual SCIP measures were independently associated with surgical infection rates. However, they did find that a composite process measure of adherence to all measures was associated with lower infection rates (14.2 vs. 6.8 per 1000 discharges [adjusted odds ratio, 0.85; 95 % confidence interval, 0.76–0.95]), suggesting that perhaps rather than the measures themselves, there are other aspects of the local environment that are associated with adherence, e.g., better coordination of care or communication among providers, that explains the lower infection rate. This study was the first to demonstrate the relationship between SCIP measure adherence and outcomes in the real world.

The research on using surgical outcomes as quality measures is robust. The development and refinement of the risk-adjusted outcomes measures within the Veterans Affairs and American College of Surgeons National Surgical Quality Improvement Program (ACS-NSQIP), is considered landmark scientific work. Ongoing work in this area continues to refine when outcomes measures offer the best approach to assessing quality. Despite having the highest degree of face validity – i.e., surgeons believe results reflect performance—measuring quality with outcomes has important limitations. It is important for surgical outcomes research to explore these limitations. For example, recent research has documented that small sample size is a key limitation of hospital- or surgeon-specific outcome measurement. Small sample size makes it difficult to achieve accurate point estimates and increases the likelihood that apparent differences in outcome reflect chance rather than true differences in care. This problem is analogous to underpowered clinical trials that lead to Type 2 errors.

For the large majority of surgical procedures, very few hospitals or surgeons have sufficient adverse events (numerators) and cases (denominators) for meaningful, procedure-specific measures of morbidity or mortality. For example, a study by our group published in the *Journal of the American Medical Association* examined seven surgical procedures, for which hospital mortality rates had been recommended as quality indicators by the Agency for Healthcare Quality and Research (AHRQ) [8]. For only one operation, coronary artery bypass graft (CABG), did the majority of U.S. hospitals perform enough cases over a 3-year period to detect with statistical confidence mortality rates at least twice the national average. For the remaining six procedures, few hospitals had sufficient caseloads to meet this low bar of statistical power. This study shed light on the problem with small sample size and highlights the importance of being thoughtful about analyzing and reporting hospital- and especially surgeon-specific outcomes. There are newer statistical modeling techniques, discussed later, that can be used to address this problem.

There are several important research tools for quality measurement. These include large database analyses, advanced statistical modeling techniques, and the concepts of risk-adjustment modeling. There are a number of large administrative or clinical databases available. For example, more than 600 hospitals across the United States participate in the ACS-NSQIP. Other large databases include the National Cancer Database, the National Trauma Database, and administrative datasets, such as national Medicare data or the Nationwide Inpatient Sample (NIS). Advanced statistical techniques, such as hierarchical modeling, are becoming increasingly important in this work. Hierarchical modeling can be used to minimize problems with small sample size (discussed above) by using empirical Bayes techniques to "adjust for reliability". Finally, risk-adjustment techniques are used to ensure that hospital outcome comparisons account for differences in patient severity of illness. It is important to point out that the use of these tools themselves is an important area of research. For example, there is ongoing debate about how comprehensive models need to be to provide adequate risk adjustment. Recent research demonstrated that more parsimonious models (5 variables vs. >20 variables) are almost as effective but require much less data collection [9].

Implementation Science

There is often a fine line between research and operational improvement initiatives when it comes to improving the quality of the care that we provide to our patients. In fact, for those of us involved in this type of research the line is often blurred. The term "quality improvement" usually applies to the operational aspect of improving care while "implementation science" is a discipline that is devoted to studying the optimal approach to organizational change and performance improvement. A landmark study by Pronovost published in the *New England Journal of Medicine* in 2006 highlights these issues [10]. Pronovost designed and implemented a checklist for placement of central lines across the state of Michigan. The authors were able to show a decrease in the mean rate of catheter-related infections from 7.7 to 2.3 per 1000 catheter-days and in fact dropping the median from 2.7 to 0 infections per 1000 catheter-days within 3 months. The results were sustained over the 18-month study period. Controversy erupted around this work when it was discovered that the IRB at Johns Hopkins did not consider this work to be human subjects research, a decision with which the federal Office for Human Research Protection (OHRP) did not agree. This highlights the importance of being clear about the goals of your work. According to OHRP, if the goal is to improve local performance than it is not research; however, if you intend to study the impact of your intervention and disseminate your results so that care can be improved more broadly, it is considered human subjects research. This distinction can be extremely challenging. The patients in Michigan clearly benefited from the intervention and the goal was to improve care at those hospitals, yet it is critical to learn from that experience so that others may achieve similar successes.

Regardless of these difficulties, the success of this study has been followed by several other high profile checklist based interventions including the Surgical Safety Checklist for intra-operative safety and the SURgical PAtient Safety System (SURPASS) checklist for the entire peri-operative period [11, 12]. Both interventions led to a documented decrease in mortality and were published in the *New England Journal of Medicine* in the last few years.

We anticipate that the fields of implementation and dissemination science (D&I) will continue to expand and grow in the coming years. There is a critical need to improve the process by which the new knowledge generated from research reaches the frontlines to implement policy and clinical practice change. It is clear that practice guidelines and clinical care pathways are not sufficient. D&I takes a scientific approach to understanding and promoting behavioral and organizational change. A pre-requisite to D&I research is that an evidence-based intervention exists that is ready for widespread adoption in practice. D&I research then aims to study this process and often involves the development of additional interventions such as toolkits that can aid providers and/or institutions in making the changes necessary to facilitate uptake of the evidence-based practice.

Patient Safety

The National Patient Safety Foundation defines patient safety as the avoidance, prevention and amelioration of adverse outcomes or injuries stemming from the processes of healthcare. Patient safety research is therefore the academic discipline dedicated to the study of these unintended negative consequences that healthcare, whether that is an individual intervention or the design of the healthcare system, can have for patients. Surgery is ripe for patient safety interventions as numerous population-based studies have repeatedly shown that surgical adverse events account for approximately half of the injuries patients encounter while in the hospital and that most of these injuries originate in the operating room. Several studies by Dr. Atul Gawande and Selwyn Rogers published in Surgery utilized a variety of techniques including analysis of closed malpractice claims and focused interviews with surgeons to identify the most common contributing factors to errors leading to injury in surgical patients [13, 14]. Carthey and deLeval, a human factors expert and a surgeon, teamed up to investigate how major and minor errors in the operating room can have significant consequences for survival following aortic switch operations, demonstrating the impact of intraoperative errors [15].

Our group uses a variety of techniques to understand patient safety and system performance in the operating room. While field observations have been traditionally used for most studies in this area, more recently the widespread availability of audiovideo (AV) capture in the operating room has replaced real-time observers. Such AV data can be used for both quantitative and qualitative analyses as well as automated video processing to study both safety and performance. As an example, we analyzed a number of complex operations and found that counter to prevailing dogma, individual practitioners were more often a source of resilience (i.e., increase prevention or mitigation of adverse events) than safety compromise. In other words, the system in the OR is quite poorly designed and the adaptability of human beings helps keep patients safe. This has major policy and educational implications, suggesting that increased standardization such as the checklist movement described above must be balanced with interventions and education to promote provider adaptability and independence [16].

Both implementation science and patient safety require a more granular approach to research than any of the other intellectual disciplines described in this chapter. The information required to understand how and why things go wrong and how they can best be improved can rarely be found in large national datasets. Studies of malpractice claims can provide larger numbers, but much of this type of work is based on point of care research. Observational field studies, focused interviews and other qualitative research techniques can provide critical information. However, quantitative assessments are also important. As described above, de Leval used statistical modeling to document the relationship between intra-operative errors and post-operative outcomes [15]. Other techniques such as statistical process control charts can help to document the results of an intervention and distinguish them from chance. Human factors engineering, cognitive psychology and organizational behavior are just a few examples of the disciplines that can provide critical tools for research in this area.

Optimizing the Healthcare Delivery System

Overview

In the context of our conceptual model, we consider the health care delivery system to represent the external factors that influence and act upon the various micro-systems of care. Aspects of the delivery system—the "macro environment"—include the workforce, payment, and the social context. Each of these elements is influenced by health policy and regulatory changes. To practicing clinicians, this environment is almost invisible. Nonetheless, it directly shapes how we function in various microsystems and how we make choices about treating patients. As a result, the delivery system has far reaching effects in health care. Despite the important influence of these external forces, health policy evaluation is rarely the focus of surgical scientists. We will consider two areas of scientific inquiry related to the delivery system: policy evaluation, and assessing the surgical workforce.

Intellectual Disciplines and Research Tools

Policy Evaluation

There are numerous national, state, and local health care policy changes each year that influence surgical practice. Oftentimes, the impact of these policies on surgical outcomes and costs are not adequately evaluated. As just one example, the Center for Medicare and Medicaid Services (CMS) issued a national coverage decision for bariatric surgery in 2006. CMS ruled that it would only reimburse for bariatric surgery performed in a Center of Excellence, as defined by criteria set forth by professional organizations. The impact of this policy is unclear. Did it improve outcomes for bariatric patients in the Medicare population? Were there spillover effects, with improved outcomes in younger patients? It is easy to undertake evaluations of such a policy and get the wrong answer. With this policy, for instance, several investigators evaluated outcomes in Medicare patients before vs. after this policy was implemented. All of these studies showed improved outcomes but they failed to account for pre-existing secular trends towards improved outcomes—i.e., they got the wrong answer.

Rigorous policy evaluation research can provide correct answers to these important questions. To evaluate this Medicare policy for bariatric surgery, we published a study in JAMA using a "difference-in-differences" analysis based on data from 3 years before and 3 years after (2004–2009) [17, 18]. This econometric method assesses the impact of a policy change **above and beyond** pre-existing trends towards improved outcomes. In this analysis, after accounting for patient factors, changes in procedure type, and preexisting time trends toward improved outcomes, we found no statistically significant improvements in outcomes after (vs. before) implementation of the policy for any complication (8.0% after vs. 7.0% before; relative risk [RR], 1.14 [95% CI, 0.95–1.33]), serious complications (3.3 vs. 3.6%, respectively; RR, 0.92 [95% CI, 0.62–1.22]), and reoperation (1.0 vs. 1.1%; RR, 0.90 [95% CI, 0.64–1.17]).

Another example of policy evaluation was conducted to evaluate pay-for-performance in the national Medicare population. Using the national Medicare database, Ryan and colleagues evaluated the impact of the Premier Hospital Incentive Demonstration [19]. This Medicare demonstration project provided up to 2% bonuses to hospitals performing in the top decile on a composite measure of process and outcome. Two surgical procedures were included, coronary artery bypass and hip replacement. Ryan also used a "difference-in-difference" analysis to adjust for secular trends in outcomes. Much like the example in bariatric surgery discussed above, this technique turned out to be important. A naïve analysis that simply looked at mortality before and after the implementation of the pay-for-performance program would have shown a significant reduction in mortality and Medicare payments. However, after accounting for pre-existing trends using the methods described above, pay-for-performance had no impact on mortality or payments. This study dampened enthusiasm for this approach and caused policymakers to rethink how they construct incentives in pay-for-performance programs.

Surgical Workforce

There is perhaps no policy issue with more divergent opinions than the adequacy of the surgical workforce [20]. On one hand, many educators and clinical leaders believe there is a severe looming shortage of surgeons. Evidence in favor of this position includes an aging population, increasing rates of surgical procedures, and the declining interest among medical students in surgical residency. On the other hand, leading policy experts believe there is more of a geographic imbalance in the workforce, with relative shortages in rural areas. Evidence in favor of this argument comes from the Dartmouth Atlas of healthcare which shows dramatic variability in the per capita surgeon workforce in the US. Experts from Dartmouth argue that it's difficult to focus on a 10% shortage when there are presently 50% differences in rates of per capita surgeons across regions of the United States. The key question, which remains unanswered, is "how many surgeons per capita is the right number?". This area of scientific study is incredibly important but understudied.

It is necessary to have a working knowledge of health policy, economics, sociology, and/or anthropology to conduct influential research in the healthcare delivery system. There are also a variety of research tools necessary to conduct research in the healthcare delivery system. Econometrics provides key tools for evaluating polices in large databases, including panel data analysis, which provides many techniques for dealing with confounding, including the difference-in-difference approach, fixed effects regression, and instrumental variable analysis. Each of these provides sophisticated analytic tools to adjust for observed and unobserved confounding factors, such as secular trends towards improvement or differences in baseline hospital performance.

At the other end of the spectrum, there are qualitative techniques from sociology and anthropology that help us understand the impact of these macro-system factors on individuals within the system. The mechanisms underlying intended and unintended consequences of changes in the delivery system can only be understood by examining the behavior and thought processes of individuals interacting with the system. Qualitative techniques include key informant interviews, focus groups, and observation, with a rigorous coding and analysis of data.

An understanding of cutting-edge health policy will help surgeons identify important policy changes, especially in the context of demonstration or pilot programs. These programs provide "natural experiments" for evaluating policy interventions. Investigators interested in this area should read *Health Affairs*, reports from the Medicare Payment Advisory Commission (MedPAC), and follow health care reform debates in Congress.

References

1. U S Department of health and human Services. Federal Coordinating Council for Comparative Effectiveness Research Report to the President and the Congress, (2009) Online.
2. Hu JC, et al. Comparative effectiveness of minimally invasive vs open radical prostatectomy. JAMA J Am Med Asso. 2009;302(14):1557–64.
3. Patient-Centered Outcomes Research Institute. PCORI Patient-Centered Outcomes Research Institute 2011–2016 [cited 2011]. Available from: http://www.pcori.org/.
4. Greenberg CC, et al. Do variations in provider discussions explain socioeconomic disparities in postmastectomy breast reconstruction? J Am Coll Surg. 2008;206(4):605–15.
5. Liu JH, et al. Disparities in the utilization of high-volume hospitals for complex surgery. JAMA. 2006;296(16):1973–80.
6. Birkmeyer JD, et al. Hospital volume and surgical mortality in the United States. N Engl J Med. 2002;346(15):1128–37.
7. Stulberg JJ, et al. Adherence to surgical care improvement project measures and the association with postoperative infections. JAMA. 2010;303(24):2479–85.
8. Dimick JB, Welch HG, Birkmeyer JD. Surgical mortality as an indicator of hospital quality: the problem with small sample size. JAMA. 2004;292(7):847–51.
9. Dimick JB, Osborne NH, Hall BL, Ko CY, Birkmeyer JD. Risk adjustment for comparing hospital quality with surgery: how many variables are needed? J Am Coll Surg. 2010;210(4):503–8.
10. Pronovost P, et al. An intervention to decrease catheter-related bloodstream infections in the ICU. N Engl J Med. 2006;355(26):2725–32.

11. Haynes AB, et al. A surgical safety checklist to reduce morbidity and mortality in a global population. N Engl J Med. 2009;360(5):491–9.
12. de Vries EN, et al. Effect of a comprehensive surgical safety system on patient outcomes. N Engl J Med. 2010;363(20):1928–37.
13. Rogers Jr SO, et al. Analysis of surgical errors in closed malpractice claims at 4 liability insurers. Surgery. 2006;140(1):25–33.
14. Gawande AA, et al. Analysis of errors reported by surgeons at three teaching hospitals. Surgery. 2003;133(6):614–21.
15. de Leval MR, et al. Human factors and cardiac surgery: a multicenter study. J Thorac Cardiovasc Surg. 2000;119(4 Pt 1):661–72.
16. Hu YY, et al. Protecting patients from an unsafe system: the etiology and recovery of intraoperative deviations in care. Ann Surg. 2012;256(2):203–10.
17. Dimick JB, et al. Bariatric surgery complications before vs after implementation of a national policy restricting coverage to centers of excellence. JAMA. 2013;309(8):792–9.
18. Dimick JB, Nicholas LH, Ryan AM, Thumma JR, Birkmeyer JD. Bariatric surgery complications before vs after implementation of a national policy restricting coverage to centers of excellence. JAMA. 2013;309(8):792–9.
19. Ryan AM. Effects of the premier hospital quality incentive demonstration on medicare patient mortality and cost. Health Serv Res. 2009;44(3):821–42.
20. Etzioni DA, et al. Getting the science right on the surgeon workforce issue. Arch Surg. 2011;146(4):381–4.

Chapter 8
Surgical Educational Research: Getting Started

Roger H. Kim

Introduction

As a result of the changing environment of medicine, which places a premium on clinical productivity, the traditional model of the surgeon/scientist with a basic science laboratory has become increasingly rare. There has been a growing recognition of the clinical educator as a viable alternative career path for advancement for academic surgeons who are unable to spend the 70–80 % of their time dedicated to research that is required for many extramural grants. In addition, publications based on surgical education research have increased in both number and quality over the past few decades. Because of this, education research has become established as a "legitimate" academic pursuit for surgeons.

However, most surgeons starting their academic career, whether at the faculty level or during their medical school or residency training, have limited exposure to surgical education research. This chapter will provide an introduction to getting started in surgical education research and will explore the rationale for pursuing education research as a career focus, discuss the challenges of such a pursuit, provide an overview of the different commonly explored topics of surgical education research, and provide guidance on how to start a surgical education research program.

R.H. Kim, M.D.
Louisiana State University Health Sciences Center – Shreveport, Shreveport, USA

Table 8.1 Benefits and challenges of surgical education research

Benefits
Low barrier to entry
Opportunities for career advancement
Opportunities for national involvement
Sense of accomplishment and gratification
Challenges
Limited funding
Limited statistical power
Academic credibility
Limited mentorship

Why Pursue Surgical Education Research?

For the purposes of this chapter, let us assume that one has chosen a career in academic surgery. What are the reasons for selecting surgical education research as the scholarly activity for one's career? A summary of both the benefits and challenges of a career in surgical education research is listed in the (Table 8.1).

Low Barrier to Entry

First and foremost, getting started in surgical education research does not present the same barriers that often exist in basic science or clinical/translational research. There are generally low start-up costs, as there is limited need for specialized laboratory equipment or reagents. With the exception of simulation-based research, which may involve some initial capital outlay, educational research can often be conducted with minimal costs.

Furthermore, the research subjects of educational studies are readily available at most academic institutions, in the form of medical students, residents, and fellows. These subjects are usually very willing to participate, making recruitment relatively straightforward compared to the recruitment of patients for clinical trials.

At many institutions, few, if any, surgeons are heavily involved in educational research. Because of this, there is often little competition for whatever departmental resources may exist to support this type of research. In addition, junior faculty are often tapped to serve as surgical educators early on, allowing for ample opportunity to "get credit twice" or "kill two birds with one stone" by leveraging administrative duties into research projects. For example, an assignment by the chair to update the surgical skills curriculum can easily be re-imagined as a chance to study the effects and outcomes of curriculum change in a pre- and post-intervention manner.

Career Advancement Opportunities

Secondly, surgical education research can provide a viable pathway to academic advancement. Within one's own institution, efforts related to student education are aligned closely with the mission of the medical school. This allows for a potential path from involvement as surgical clerkship director to administrative positions under the dean of the medical school, such as associate dean of student affairs, overseeing the entire body of medical students. Within the department of surgery, residency program directors and fellowship directors are considered key personnel, critical to the overall success of the department. Although the Accreditation Council for Graduate Medical Education (ACGME) requires that individuals have served at least 5 years as a faculty member prior to appointment as a program director, there is no such requirement for associate program directors: junior faculty can start as associate program directors and progress to program directors later in their careers. In addition, some departments have created positions such as vice-chair of education or vice-chair of academic affairs; these individuals often oversee all the educational efforts of the department and represent an avenue for surgical educators to enter senior leadership positions. Some medical schools have an associate dean for graduate medical education, providing another option for advancement.

Opportunity for National Involvement

As mentioned above, there are an ever increasing number of organizations and forums that provide opportunities for both academic dissemination of surgical educational research findings and for involvement/advancement within these associations. The Association for Academic Surgery (AAS), the Society of University Surgeons (SUS), the American College of Surgeons (ACS), the Association for Surgical Education (ASE), the Association of Program Directors in Surgery (APDS), and the Association of American Medical Colleges (AAMC) are among the many organizations that have meetings in which education-based projects can be presented. These organizations also have affiliations with journals that accept surgical education manuscripts for publication, including the *Journal of Surgical Research*, *Surgery*, the *Journal of the American College of Surgeons*, the *American Journal of Surgery*, the *Journal of Surgical Education*, and *Academic Medicine*. In addition, each of these associations has opportunities to get involved on a national level through a variety of committees related to surgical education [1].

Sense of Accomplishment/Gratification

Educational research offers ample opportunity for rapid implementation of research findings into real-world applications. Changes in curriculum can often be made within a single academic year cycle. This is in contrast to the generally slower turn-around time for basic science or even clinical research findings to enter clinical practice. This allows for a more immediate gratification for the surgical educator, in which an opportunity for improvement is noticed, studied in a research setting, and then implemented into the curriculum in relatively quick fashion.

Finally, many of us in academic surgery first considered a career in academics because of the teaching aspect. Since surgical education research is most often performed in conjunction with, or as an adjunct to, teaching sessions with medical students, residents or fellows, the sense of accomplishment that comes from the academic achievement is often enhanced by a similar sense of accomplishment that comes from the successful training of those learners under our tutelage. As with any scholarly activity, one is likely to be more productive if the academic pursuit is aligned with one's passions and interests.

Challenges of Surgical Education Research

As one contemplates going into surgical education research, it is important to recognize some of the challenges that exist in this field. While not insurmountable obstacles, awareness of these challenges is critical in order to be successful in surgical education research.

Limited Funding

Perhaps the biggest challenge is the relatively limited extramural research funding earmarked for surgical education [2]. The funding opportunities that do exist will be discussed in greater detail later in this chapter. However, most surgical education research, especially early on, is conducted without funding from extramural grants.

Limited Statistical Power

While research subjects are often readily available for surgical educational research projects, their numbers can be sometimes limited. This is particularly true for research focused on surgical residents, as few programs have more than five categorical residents per post-graduate year (PGY). This can lead to inadequately powered studies due to small sample size. Longitudinal studies may partially alleviate this limitation, but at the expense of a longer study period. The use of multi-institutional studies is perhaps the best method to deal with this issue, but introduces problems of logistics. Because of the larger size of most medical school classes compared to surgical residency programs, research projects focused on medical students are generally less prone to this limitation.

Academic Credibility

While the reputation of education research has improved dramatically, there still remain some academic surgeons who persist in not considering it "serious research" compared to basic science or clinical research. The reason for this reputation is multifactorial and beyond the scope of this chapter to explore in depth. Suffice it to say that an academic surgeon who chooses to pursue a career in surgical education research should be prepared to deal with colleagues who may view their projects with a lower level of respect than they would for projects in other research disciplines.

Limited Mentorship

While some departments of surgery have established impressive programs devoted to surgical education research with multiple experienced investigators, most departments have limited, if any, significant experience in surgical education research. Academic surgeons who are seeking to start a career in education research often find themselves as the only faculty member in their department doing so. As a result, there is often limited mentorship available within the department. Methods of seeking out alternate models of mentorship for surgical education research will be discussed later in this chapter.

Topics of Surgical Education Research

There are several different methods by which surgical education research can be categorized. One common approach is to categorize by research design methodology, i.e., quantitative vs. qualitative. Another approach is to categorize by subject matter. It is this latter approach that will be used in defining some of the common domains of surgical education research [3–5]. This list is neither exhaustive nor exclusive, as many research projects may span more than one of these categories, and some may not be easily be classified into any particular category. Nevertheless, this list can serve as a starting point for an investigator starting out in surgical education research.

Simulation

The amount of research in this category has increased significantly in recent years, in part due to advances in simulation technology. While much of simulation research as it relates to surgical education has been focused on technical skills, particularly in regards to minimally-invasive surgery, simulation can also encompass non-technical skills and other ACGME competencies, such as communication skills and professionalism. The emphasis of technical skills simulation in surgical education research is likely to remain, however, given the emphasis on teaching efficiency in the era of duty-hour restrictions. An area of significant research interest is on the transferability of simulation-based training into the real-world operative setting and whether simulation can improve patient outcomes [3].

Assessment

This category can encompass both medical student and resident assessment and can include self-assessments, performance evaluations by faculty, or multiple-choice question tests such as the American Board of Surgery In-Training Examination (ABSITE). Recently, technical skills assessment has become a growing focus within this category. Objective Structured Assessment of Technical Skills (OSATS), the Fundamentals of Laparoscopic Surgery (FLS) test, and Global Operative Assessment of Laparoscopic Skills (GOALS) are among the primary examples of technical skills assessment methods. An important component of this category of research is the development of new assessment tools and the establishment of their reliability and validity. This is of increasing importance with the recent implementation of the ACGME General Surgery Milestones Project, as many of the milestones do not yet have assessment instruments that are both valid and reliable [3–5].

Curriculum and Teaching

Curriculum development can be applied to medical student education in the preclinical years and the clinical clerkships, as well as surgical resident training. Teaching can encompass both basic science and clinical science teaching. Research within this domain can include the effects of new surgical curricula or novel instructional methods on the acquisition of knowledge by trainees. The Surgical Council on Resident Education (SCORE) general surgery curriculum serves as a key framework for future research in this area, at least as it applies to the ACGME core competencies of medical knowledge and patient care [4–5].

Team Training

Much of surgical education research in the past has focused on learners as individuals. However, there is a growing recognition of the need to focus on team training. Teamwork directly relates to the ACGME core competencies of professionalism, interpersonal and communication skills, and system-based practice. Team training-based research projects often incorporate simulated patient care scenarios and are frequently conducted across multiple disciplines, such as anesthesia, emergency medicine, surgical technicians, and nursing [3].

Starting a Surgical Education Research Program

There are a few issues that are unique to surgical education research that must be taken into consideration when starting a research program. These include the assembly of the research team, the identification of possible funding sources, and the various forums available for the publication and dissemination of research findings.

The Surgical Education Research Team

While a growing number of surgical educators pursue advanced degrees in education, most investigators will require assistance from collaborators with specialized expertise. A research team comprised of experts from multiple disciplines can greatly enhance the quality, feasibility and success of a surgical education research program. A medical educator or educational specialist, who usually possesses a Master's or Ph. D. in education or an Ed. D., can greatly assist in understanding the educational theory that most surgical investigators have had little exposure to previously. While few departments of surgery employ a medical educator directly, many medical schools have such a role within the dean's office; such an individual may be able to serve as a mentor in this capacity for the surgical education researcher. Alternatively, this type of expertise may be sought through a university's school of education.

As is the case with most other research endeavors, the involvement of a statistician can be extremely helpful in both study design and analysis. A nurse educator or simulation expert can be helpful in the implementation and execution of different educational interventions. A qualitative researcher is critical if qualitative research studies will be part of the program, as very few surgeons will have any experience with the nuances of this type of research design. Partnering with an educator with expertise in survey design can be extremely valuable for similar reasons. While it may not be feasible or necessary to have all of these roles filled within a surgical education research program, a research team with a diverse skill set is required to be successful. Depending on the situation, individuals may be able to serve in multiple roles.

Mentorship within surgical education research deserves a special mention. There is a relative paucity of people qualified to be mentors in this field, especially in comparison to other domains of academic surgery. Often, the identification of a suitable mentor will require looking outside one's own institution. This is where involvement on a national level through organizations such as the AAS, ACS, ASE, or the APDS can be of great help. The Surgical Education Research Fellowship (SERF), sponsored by the ASE, is an example of an organized effort to pair nationally recognized leaders in surgical education with mentees pursuing the completion of a specific project. One can also take advantage of having a team of mentors, each with expertise in different facets of surgical education research. Any of the aforementioned members of the research team can also, given the proper circumstances, serve as a potential mentor for the aspiring surgical educator.

Funding Opportunities

As alluded to earlier, there are extremely limited funds dedicated to medical education research. Most of the traditional extramural sources for research funding, such as the National Institutes of Health (NIH), do not have specific funding categories earmarked for medical education research, although some projects may be eligible for funding if they fall under an appropriate program. However, the reality is that the vast majority of published research is not formally funded and relies on departmental and institutional support, particularly in the early phases.

Perhaps the best example for a funding opportunity specific to surgical education is the Center for Excellence in Surgical Education, Research and Training (CESERT) grants program. Developed by the ASE Foundation, this program supports innovation in surgical education research in North America. Priority is given to ASE members, but non-members can apply in collaboration with, or with the endorsement of an ASE member.

The Stemmler Medical Education Research Fund, established by the National Board of Medical Examiners (NBME), supports research for undergraduate, graduate, or continuing medical education. Medical schools accredited through the Liaison Committee on Medical Education (LCME) or the American Osteopathic Association (AOA) are eligible to apply for this program.

The AAS Roslyn Faculty Research Award provides early career support to junior faculty AAS members who are within 5 years of completion of training and have not yet been promoted to the rank of Associate Professor. This award is not specific to surgical education research. The AAS also funds research awards for medical students and residents or fellows. The ACS Faculty Research Fellowships and the Society of American Gastrointestinal and Endoscopic Surgeons (SAGES) Career Development Award also target surgeons within 5 years of completion of training.

Among federal funding sources, the American Educational Research Association (AERA), supported by the National Science Foundation (NSF), provides research grants for educational projects involving the analysis of at least one large-scale, federal agency-supported data set. The NSF also funds research through its Directorate for Education and Human Resources (EHR) through a variety of programs, some of which may be applicable to education research. The Agency for Healthcare Research and Quality (AHRQ) has offered research grants aimed at improving patient safety through simulation. The Health Resources and Services

Administration (HRSA) of the Department of Health and Human Services also may provide funding for education research.

The four regional groups of the Association of the American Medical Colleges (AAMC) Group on Educational Affairs (GEA) each provide funding opportunities for medical education research projects within their respective regions: the Central, the Northeastern, the Southern, and the Western. The Society for Academic Continuing Medical Education (SACME) offers the Phil R. Manning Research Award in Continuing Medical Education to support research in the field of continuing medical education and professional development.

Some charitable foundations offer grants in medical education research. The Josiah Macy Jr. Foundation supports research in the areas of interprofessional education and teamwork, new curriculum content, new models for clinical education, education for the care of underserved populations, and career development in health professions education. The Arnold P. Gold Foundation sponsors the Picker Gold Challenge Grants in Residency Training, which support research on patient-centered care initiatives within graduate medical education. The Arthur Vining Davis Foundations have also supported health care education projects in the past.

Finally, educational research funding can sometimes be obtained through institutional support through the medical school dean's office, state funding resources (particularly for public medical schools), or through industry support. A summary of the various resources for funding and the related websites are provided in Table 8.2 [2].

Forums for Publication/Presentation

There are a variety of options for publishing or presenting surgical education research findings. Abstracts can be submitted to academic conferences; the primary focus of such meetings can either be surgical or education. The Academic Surgical Congress is jointly hosted by the AAS and the SUS and represents the largest annual meeting of academic surgeons in the world. This combined meeting accepts surgical education research abstracts for presentation and includes a dedicated Education Plenary Session. The ACS Clinical Congress is the largest meeting of surgeons in the world and hosts the Scientific Forum, which includes education as one of its presentation categories. The ACS also hosts the annual meeting of ACS-Accredited Education Institutes (AEI), which is focused on simulation-based education. Surgical Education Week, a combined meeting of the ASE, the APDS, and the Association of Residency Coordinators in Surgery (ARCS), is focused solely on surgical education research. The ASE accepts abstracts in all realms of surgical education, while the APDS focuses on surgical education primarily as it pertains to residency training. The AAMC GEA hosts an annual Research in Medical Education (RIME) Conference in conjunction with the annual meeting of the AAMC, during which educational research abstracts are presented. The regional AACM GEA meetings also have annual meetings that offer educational research sessions. The

Table 8.2 Grant programs and funding opportunities in surgical education research

Federal agencies	Website
American Education Research Association (AERA)	http://www.aera.net/
National Science Foundation (NSF) – Directorate for Education and Human Resources (EHR)	http://www.nsf.gov/dir/index.jsp?org=EHR
Agency for Healthcare Research and Quality (AHRQ)	http://www.ahrq.gov/
Department of Health and Human Services – Health Resources and Services Administration (HRSA)	http://www.hrsa.gov/
Professional societies/associations	
Association for Surgical Education (ASE) – Center for Excellence in Surgical Education, Research and Training (CESERT)	https://surgicaleducation.com/cesert-grants
National Board of Medical Examiners (NBME) – Stemmler Medical Education Research Fund	http://www.nbme.org/research/stemmler.html
Association for Academic Surgery (AAS) – Roslyn Faculty Research Award	http://www.aasurg.org/awards/award_roslyn.php
American College of Surgeons (ACS) – Faculty Research Fellowships	https://www.facs.org/member-services/scholarships/research/acsfaculty
Society of American Gastrointestinal and Endoscopic Surgeons (SAGES) – Career Development Award	http://www.sages.org/projects/sages-career-development-award/
Association of the American Medical Colleges (AAMC) – Group on Educational Affairs (GEA)	https://www.aamc.org/members/gea/
Society for Academic Continuing Medical Education (SACME) – Phil R. Manning Research Award in Continuing Medical Education	http://www.sacme.org/SACME_Grants
Charitable foundations	
Josiah Macy Jr. Foundation	http://macyfoundation.org/apply
Arnold P. Gold Foundation – Picker Gold Challenge Grants in Residency Training	http://humanism-in-medicine.org/programs/picker-gold-challenge-grants-for-residency-training/
Arthur Vining Davis Foundations	http://www.avdf.org/Grants/GrantsOverview.aspx
Other	
Industry partners	
State funding	
Institutional support	
Departmental support	

Table 8.3 Professional societies related to surgical education

Professional society/association	Meeting	Affiliated journal
Association for Academic Surgery (AAS)	Academic Surgical Congress	*Journal of Surgical Research*
Society of University Surgeons (SUS)	Academic Surgical Congress	*Surgery*
Association for Surgical Education (ASE)	Surgical Education Week	*American Journal of Surgery*
Association of Program Directors in Surgery (APDS)	Surgical Education Week	*Journal of Surgical Education*
American College of Surgeons (ACS)	Clinical Congress	*Journal of the American College of Surgeons*
ACS – Accredited Education Institutes (AEI)	Annual AEI Consortium Meeting	*Surgery*
Association of American Medical Colleges (AAMC)	AAMC Annual Meeting	*Academic Medicine*
Society of American Gastrointestinal and Endoscopic Surgeons (SAGES)	SAGES Annual Meeting	*Surgical Endoscopy*

SAGES Annual Meeting accepts abstracts in education, particularly related to minimally invasive surgery or endoscopy.

Many of these sponsoring organizations have partnerships with journals to which manuscripts based on accepted abstracts may be submitted for publication. A list of these societies, their meetings, and the affiliated journals is provided in Table 8.3.

Finally, a non-traditional method of publishing work in surgical education research is MedEdPortal, a free publication services provided by the AAMC. MedEdPortal serves as a clearinghouse of peer-reviewed health education tools and as a forum for the exchange of educational resources.

Conclusion

With proper recognition of the issues and challenges unique to surgical education research, an understanding of the research topics within the field, and the thoughtful assembly of a dedicated team, surgical education research can be a highly rewarding and fulfilling focus for an academic career in surgery.

References

1. Pugh CM, Sippel RS. Success in academic surgery: developing a career in surgical education. London: Springer; 2013.
2. Capella J, Kasten SJ, Steinemann S, Torbeck L. Guide for research in surgical education. Woodbury: Cine-Med; 2010.

3. Wohlauer MV, George B, Lawrence PF, Pugh CM, Van Eaton EG, DaRosa D. Review of influential articles in surgical education: 2002–2012. J Grad Med Educ. 2013;5(2):219–26.
4. Derossis AM, DaRosa DA, Dutta S, Dunnington GL. A ten-year analysis of surgical education research. Am J Surg. 2000;180(1):58–61.
5. Rotgans JI. The themes, institutions, and people of medical education research 1988–2010: content analysis of abstracts from six journals. Adv Health Sci Educ Theory Pract. 2012;17(4):515–27.

Chapter 9
Translational Research and New Approaches: Genomics, Proteomics, and Metabolomics

David P. Foley

In the current era of practicing medicine, it has become increasingly more difficult for surgeons to become successful researchers. As Dr. Craig Kent summarized in his Keynote Address at the Fundamental Surgical Research Course in 2009, the challenges that surgeons face are numerable. Surgery requires continual practice and maintenance of sound surgical technique by doing surgery, a circumstance that does not allow for lengthy periods of protected time. Institutional culture disfavors research in surgery. Due to decreased reimbursements from third-party payors and Medicare, many administrators would rather see the surgeon generating clinical revenue by performing surgery instead of doing experiments in the laboratory. At the divisional level, one may be frowned upon in asking for financial divisional support to support a research program while the partners shoulder his or her clinical load. In many areas of surgery, "medical competitors" perform similar types of research. However, medical competitors do not suffer the same limitations in developing their research programs, as do surgeons.

Another challenge facing surgeons is that sustainable research requires funding and sources of funding have decreased over recent years. Success rates for attaining funding from the National Institutes of Health have also decreased. Based on data from the NIH, the success rate of for R01-equivalent grants has decreased from 31 % in 1998 to 22 % in 2010. In fiscal year 2015 the success rates for R01 funding ranged between 11.8 and 28.8 % depending on the institute or center. The vast majority (68 %) of the institutes had success rates below 20 % (https://report.nih.gov/success_rates). The average age of receiving a R01 grant increased from 39 in 1990 to 43 in 2007. In addition, basic science technology has become significantly

D.P. Foley, M.D.
Department of Surgery, Division of Organ Transplantation, University of Wisconsin School of Medicine and Public Health, H4/766 Clinical Science Center, 600 Highland Ave, Madison, WI 53792-7375, USA

more complex in recent years making it more challenging for the surgical scientist to stay up-to-date while maintaining a clinical surgical practice.

Fortunately, there has been an influx of other research opportunities for surgeons that are more closely related to patient disease states and outcomes. One of those areas that continue to evolve is translational research. Translational research involves identifying and defining a clinical problem at the bedside, developing a hypothesis that can be tested in the laboratory setting, and then completing the loop by bringing those research findings back to the clinical setting for testing and improvement in clinical care. It focuses on directly linking laboratory discoveries and clinical care. Some examples include (1) the evaluation of biopsies from donor human livers with microarrays to determine if a specific expression profile predicts allograft failure or other complications after liver transplantation; (2) the identification of diagnostic biomarkers for human hepatocellular carcinoma by using mass spectroscopy; or (3) the determination of whether doxycycline administration reduces protease expression in human aortic aneurysm tissue.

In 2005 the National Cancer Institute (NCI) established the Translational Research Working Group (TRWG) to conduct a discussion with a broader cancer research community and develop recommendations about how the NCI can best organize its investment to further translational research. The group defined translational research as research that "transforms scientific discoveries arising from laboratory, clinical, or population studies into clinical applications to reduce cancer incidence, morbidity, and mortality." Those participating in translational research will form the bridge between the "bench and the bedside." For instance, the discovery of novel gene targets, a promising molecule, or a candidate protein biomarker of a specific a disease identified in the basic science laboratory can lead to increased partnerships and collaboration with government, industry, or academia. It can also lead more quickly to intervention development and Phase I or II clinical trials (NCI TRWG www.cancer.gov/trwg).

Why is translational research a viable career choice for aspiring academic surgical scientists? One reason is the fact that as surgeons we perform surgery to remove tumors, to treat organ failure, and remove organs with intractable inflammatory disease. We are unique in that we are able to see pathology in the human *in vivo* setting and correlate these intraoperative findings with clinical symptoms, signs and postoperative outcomes. With adequate informed consent from the patient, we are able to safely biopsy organs, and correlate clinical and intraoperative findings with molecular and protein analyses from the biopsy tissue. We have access to tumor bank tissue, and analysis of that tissue is another viable area of research where one can study molecular signatures that may impact response to therapy and overall patient outcomes. Opportunities have also expanded to include the use of clinical databases whereby both retrospective and prospective analyses are performed to answer patient-related research questions. In addition, the use of animal surgical models that are similar to clinical situations allows for the testing of novel treatment modalities for the treatment of disease.

Recognizing the importance of transforming translational research even further, the NIH established the National Center for Advancing Translational Sciences

(NCATS) in 2012. The center was established in order to transform translational research and decrease the time that it takes to get new effective therapies to patients. There are multiple programs within NCATS that provide funding opportunities for translational researchers. One of those includes the Clinical and Translational Science Award (CTSA) Program that was initially launched in 2006. The program supports a national consortium of medical research institutions designed to transform how biomedical research is conducted. The goals are to speed the translation of laboratory discoveries into treatments for patients, to engage communities in clinical research efforts, and to train a new generation of clinical and translational researchers. Currently there are 55 institutions that are part of the CTSA consortium including 28 states and the District of Columbia. More information regarding NCATS Programs are available on their website (ncats.nih.gov/programs.html).

In addition, the NIH has increased the emphasis of clinical significance in grant proposals. Historically, basic science grant applications that resulted in funding could focus on cellular and molecular pathways and mechanisms without overemphasizing a potential transitional impact on clinical outcomes in the near future. There is now a shift towards a greater emphasis on clarifying how a research proposal addresses an important problem or a critical barrier to patient care. Studying human tissue samples and correlating these findings with disease states or treatment for a given disease allows for direct application to clinical care.

There are multiple new technologies that have been developed over recent years to study the human body's response to disease at the cellular level. These findings can be correlated with clinical outcomes and subsequently used to predict response to a specific therapy or simply to identify a novel biomarker for a particular disease. Some of these strategies include genomics, proteomics, and metabolomics. These technologies allow for the molecular examination of tissue or blood to unravel the basic biological responses to disease. The remainder of this chapter will focus on each of these strategies and various examples of how this technology can lead to a better understanding of the body's response to multiple disease states.

Genomics

Genomics involves the study of organisms' genes including the determination of the entire DNA sequence. Complete genomes have been developed for many organisms including humans. Genomics can be divided into either structural or functional genomics. Structural genomics involves the characterization of the physical nature of whole genomes, and corresponds to the genetic background of organisms. Using high-throughput technologies that allow for the simultaneous determination of a large number of components from a clinical sample, one can evaluate the variation of DNA sequence within a population. This enables the systematic study of disease-correlated genomic variations.

Biological variations can vary from a single base change termed a single nucleotide polymorphism (SNP), to small insertions or deletions of sequence called indels, to large-scale chromosomal translocations. In some instances individual mutations can produce a disease state as is seen in sickle cell anemia where a single base change in the β chain of hemoglobin (adenine to thymine), causes the replacement of glutamine with valine. Huntington's disease is caused by an expansion of the polyglutamine repeat (CAG) in the gene that encodes Huntington protein. The Philadelphia Chromosome is the result of a wholesale translocation in chromosomes 9 and 22, resulting in the production of a constitutively active tyrosine kinase that can lead to chronic myelogenous leukemia.

It is more common that a genomic variation is found to correlate with increased susceptibility to a given disease. First a specific genomic variant is identified in an individual with a disease. When the same variant is identified in another individual without evidence of the disease, the SNPs can be tested for association with susceptibility to a variety of diseases. When the frequencies of the genotype are compared in populations of cases and controls, a higher frequency in patients with the disease is thought to be sufficient evidence that the genetic variation is associated with increased risk of disease. One example is the mutation in the BRCA1 and BRCA2 gene. Women with both mutations have an 80 % lifetime risk of breast cancer compared to 12 % lifetime risk in the general population.

One example demonstrating the rapid translation of preclinical molecular findings in genomic studies into the clinic has been seen in ALK (anaplastic lymphoma kinase) gene inhibition in non-small cell lung cancer (NSCLC). ALK encodes a tyrosine kinase normally expressed only in neuronal cells. In a rare subset of anaplastic large cell lymphomas, interstitial deletion and inversion within chromosome 2p result in fusion of the N-terminal portion of the protein encoded by the echinoderm microtubule-associated protein-like 4 (ELM4) gene with the intracellular portion of the ALK receptor tyrosine kinase. While genetic alterations involving ALK have been seen in other malignancies, thus far, the ELM4-ALK fusion gene appears unique to NSCLC. In less than 3 years after these findings, studies of ALK inhibition yielded dramatic results in patients with NSCLC. In a pretreated population that generally has a 10 % response rate to conventional chemotherapy, treatment with the oral ALK inhibitor, crizotinib, yielded an overall response rate of 55 % and an estimated 6-month, progression-free survival rate of 72 % [1].

Gene-Expression Profiling

Functional genomics involves the overall patterns of gene expression and the targets of this research are RNA, proteins, and metabolites. Functional genomics allows the detection of genes that are turned on and off at a given time based on environmental factors. Transcriptomics consists of the study of all transcribed mRNA species at a given time. Multiplex oligonucleotide or complementary DNA microarrays are platforms that can be used to determine mRNA abundance of hundreds to thousands of genes simultaneously. The principles of these technologies involve the following. Oligonucleotide or complimentary DNAs (cDNAs) for specific mRNA species are immobilized on a surface (glass slide, or nylon membrane). The target mRNA is isolated from the sample of interest, converted to cDNA, labeled, and allowed to hybridize to the oligonucleotides or cDNA fixed to the solid surface. The intensity of hybridization on each probe is proportional to the gene expression level.

To perform array experiments, one needs the probes to detect the RNA, reproducible and sensitive techniques for quantification of RNA levels, and standardization procedures and databases for analysis. Array methods differ based on which probes are used (cDNA or oligonucleotides), the technology used to fix the probes to the solid surface probes, and the labeling technologies for the mRNA targets. When changes of mRNA abundance are identified and they are small in number, the microarray findings can be validated by using real-time polymerase chain reaction (PCR). PCR is more sensitive and is cheaper than using microarrays when smaller numbers of genes are studied. The two techniques are usually used in parallel fashion to validate the findings.

The most difficult aspect of employing microarray technology is not the acquisition of the data but rather the analysis. While a detailed discussion of statistical analytical methods used in genome wide studies is beyond the limitations of this chapter, a few analytical techniques will be discussed. Clustering is a data mining technique used to group genes having similar expression patterns. Hierarchical clustering and k-means clustering are widely used techniques in microarray analysis. The concept is such that genes of similar function are co-expressed to produce a specific phenotype. Hierarchical clustering is a statistical method for finding relatively homogenous clusters of similarly expressed genes. This clustering consists of two separate phases. A distance matrix containing all of the pair-wise distances between the genes is calculated. Pearson's correlation or Spearman's correlation are often used to estimate dissimilarities among genetic clusters.

Analyses are also termed either as supervised or unsupervised. Unsupervised analyses involve analyzing the most differentially expressed genes that are clustered to look for patterns. In supervised analysis, the most commonly used analysis, samples are pre-grouped using existing knowledge and then they are clustered and analyzed. For example, samples are grouped by good or poor prognosis and then genes are clustered. This approach identifies genes that are potentially linked to prognosis in a training set.

A commonly used statistical method for the analysis of microarrays is Significance Analysis of Microarrays (SAM) that was adapted by Tusher et.al. [2] SAM identifies genes with statistically significant changes in expression by assimilating a set of gene-specific t-tests. Each gene is given a score on the basis of its change in gene expression relative to the standard deviation of repeated measurements for that gene. Genes with a score greater than a pre-defined threshold are deemed potentially significant. The percentage of such genes identified by chance is the false discovery rate (FDR). In other words, the FDR is the proportion of genes that were wrongly identified by chance as being significant. It is calculated by dividing the median of the number of falsely called genes by the number of genes called significant. In addition, if a preliminary set of expression data are available, SAM can also estimate the number of microarray chips required to reach a defined level of significance.

There are two major areas where functional genomics can impact medicine. One is by identifying molecular markers or differentially expressed genes that may be important in biological functions as their expression differs based on environmental and genetic factors. The other application that is potentially more powerful is the ability to identify a signature profile that can be used as a detailed molecular phenotype.

These predictors could be complemented in the future with changes in structural genetic variations that are identified at the DNA level. With this technology researchers who study trauma biology and sepsis can develop molecular signatures for inflamed tissues and specific cell populations. This technology is currently being used to characterize the progress of disease in patients with trauma, burns, and sepsis. Applications can also extend to tumor biology and identifying those patients who may respond to treatment better than others. In solid organ transplantation the changes in gene expression in donor organs can be correlated with outcomes for a given recipient. These findings can assist the transplant community in determining which recipients should receive a given organ to yield the greatest benefit. Gene expression may also reflect the environmental past to which a patient may have been exposed and the impacts of those changes can be correlated with clinical signs and symptoms.

Gene expression in kidney transplant biopsies can identify which kidneys are more likely to end up in early graft failure despite no changes seen on histologic analysis. In a recent study, Modena et al. analyzed gene expression profiles of 234 kidney allograft biopsies in order to assess which kidneys with interstitial fibrosis and tubular atrophy (IFTA) seen on biopsy were more likely to lead to future graft loss. They identified a subset of kidney allografts with IFTA but without histologic evidence of inflammation that did in fact have ongoing immune mediated injury or chronic rejection. These molecular biopsy profiles correlated with future graft loss in IFTA samples without inflammation [3]. This information can lead to more aggressive treatment of subclinical inflammation and improved long term graft survival in kidney transplant recipients.

Some centers have developed comprehensive genomic programs for a specific disease process in order to define novel genetic therapeutic strategies that may work in conjunction with surgical approaches to improve long-term outcomes. Through collaborative efforts at Baylor College of Medicine, researchers have established a genomic program for the study of hepatocellular carcinoma (HCC) in order to improve both patient and allograft survival after undergoing either liver resection or liver transplantation for HCC. They have established an effective biobanking protocol and after adequate tissue is confirmed by independent pathologists, genomic sequencing is performed. Their genomic sequencing includes whole genome sequencing, whole exome sequencing, gene-specific analysis, gene expression, and epigenetic analysis. After all data are analyzed, and true genetic mutations are identified, it is hoped that that they will identify those genetic modifications that are pivotal to HCC progression so they can prevent, stop the growth, or shrink the disease. Therapies can then be targeted to patients with specific genomic characteristics [4].

Proteomics

Proteomics is the large-scale global analysis of proteins. While genomics seeks to sequence the genes and transcriptomics seeks to understand the expression of all of genes, proteomics seeks to identify all of the proteins of the proteome. The general platform for proteomic research for the identification of novel biomarkers of disease involves the following. Proteins are extracted from biological samples and a matched control. The proteins are enzymatically digested into peptides; the peptides are ionized and then introduced into the mass spectrometer. Mass spectrometry (MS) yields the mass of the peptide whereas tandem mass spectrometry (MS/MS) yields fragment masses for sequencing. The proteins need to be digested because the majority of the MS instruments cannot yield sequence data on whole proteins. Once the MS and MS/MS data are obtained, the peptide is identified by comparing its parent mass and sequence against a database, such as *in silico* virtual digest of all of the proteins in the proteome. The virtual fragment peptides from those virtual peptides that match the mass of the parent peptide within a certain tolerance are compared against the real fragment ions obtained from the MS/MS stage. From this comparison, a statistical probability is generated which reflects the likelihood that the virtual and real peptides are the same.

One of the difficulties with proteomics is the challenge of identifying all proteins in a given sample when some may be more abundant than others. Since the mass spectrometer can only perform MS/MS to obtain sequence information on one peptide at a time, the likelihood of sequencing a low abundant protein is very low. Therefore, the peptides need to be separated before they are introduced into the mass spectrometer. The most common way of doing this is with a high-performance liquid chromatography (HPLC) coupled directly to the mass spectrometer. This technique is commonly referred to as LC MS/MS. In some instances two-dimensional HPLC separation is coupled to electrospray ionization and mass spectroscopy (ESI-MS). Typically, the first dimension is performed "offline" in which the HPLC is not connected to the MS and instead the eluting proteins or peptides are collected in fractions. Those collected fractions are then run individually in the second dimension that is most commonly a reverse phase HPLC separation that is coupled directly to the mass spectrometer. The advantages of this technique are increased sampling depth, increased ability to detect low abundant proteins, and a higher yield of total protein identifications [5].

Another technique of identifying the quantity of a protein in a given biological sample is the Luminex 100 xMAP (Multi-Analyte Profiling) System (Austin, TX). This has been used to identify cytokine levels in human plasma when assessing the systemic inflammatory state in patients undergoing lower extremity revascularization [6]. This bead-based assay system is a flow cytometric analysis using novel fluorescent beads that are covalently linked to antibodies specific for individual analytes. By coupling the specificity of antibody-based capture of specific cytokines using chromophore-labeled antibodies with flow cytometric analyses, the analytical system can multiplex the analysis of theoretically an unlimited number of cytokines simultaneously from a single sample. The Luminex technology simultaneously identifies the quantity of a given analyte, as well as its identity. Similar technology has become the gold standard for the detection and identification of deleterious alloantibodies of a kidney recipient to a specific kidney donor. The specific proteomic analytical technique that is chosen usually depends on the expertise of the collaborative team.

The introduction of peptide analysis by mass spectrometry in combination with bioinformatics for data processing has revolutionized the field of proteomics. There are multiple potential applications of proteomics to clinical medicine. These techniques can allow for protein sequencing, relative protein quantification, post-translational modifications (e.g., glycosylation or phosphorylation), protein-protein interactions and the identification of biomarkers for a given disease. Although the development of the proteomic field has lagged behind that of genomics, there are an increasing number of published studies demonstrating important clinical applications of these techniques.

In a preliminary proteomic study, Tweedle et al. studied the levels of heat shock protein 27 (HSP27) in colorectal cancer samples. The expression of HSP27 in a cohort of 404 patients with colorectal cancer with a predominantly poor prognosis was characterized. HSP27 levels in diagnostic rectal biopsies were compared with matched surgical samples to determine whether changes in expression occurred in the time between biopsy and surgery and to investigate whether preoperative radiation therapy affected expression. The authors found that HSP27 overexpression was strongly associated with poor-cancer-specific survival in rectal cancer but not in colon cancer in those with a poor prognosis. HSP27 levels remained unchanged in the majority of cases between diagnostic biopsies and matched surgical controls, regardless of whether patients had undergone preoperative radiotherapy. The authors concluded that HSP27 is an independent marker of poor outcome in rectal cancer and its expression is not affected by neoadjuvant radiotherapy. This study can lead to future studies to evaluate whether HSP27 levels should be considered as a stratification factor for the treatment of rectal cancer [7].

In another translational research study Ren et al. performed a two dimensional analysis of human hepatocellular carcinoma (HCC) line, HepG2, and an immortal hepatic cell line, LO2. They identified that phosphoglycerate mutase 1 (PGAM1) was markedly upregulated in the HepG2 line compared to controls. This finding led to determining the role of PGAM1 in patients with HCC. Immunohistochemistry (IHC) was performed on excised HCC specimens. Weak IHC staining for PGAM1 correlated with a 5-year patient survival of 55.6% compared to 18.2% in patients with tumors that demonstrated strong PGAM1 staining. In addition, shRNAs-mediated repression of PGAM1 expression resulted in significant inhibition in liver cancer cell growth both *in vitro* and *in vivo* [8]. Findings from this study that "translated" laboratory findings into the clinical setting may lead to novel therapies targeting PGAM1 in the setting of HCC.

More recently, proteomics has been used to identify urinary proteins that are related to bladder cancer. In this analysis biomarker candidates in the secreted proteins derived from bladder cancer cell lines were screened and subsequently verified in the urine of patients with cancer. Differential proteins were then defined using two-dimensional electrophoresis and isobaric tags for relative and absolute quantitation (iTRAQ) coupled with LC MS/MS. After identifying a total of 700 proteins that were secreted from tumor cell lines, the authors identified ten differential urine proteins linked to bladder cancer. Receiver operating characteristic analysis revealed the combination of CO3 and LDHB as more sensitive as the cancer indicators. This study will lead to future studies aimed at biomarker validation [9].

Another application for the use of proteomics is in the identification of novel biomarkers in the setting of traumatic brain injury (TBI). TBI has received increased publicity recently due to its high incidence among disabled soldiers returning from both Iraq and Afghanistan. In addition, TBI has also impacted both amateur and professional athletics as physicians struggle to determine when players, who sustain significant concussions, can return to full contact. The ability to diagnose the severity of TBI is challenging when relying solely on clinical parameters. Early appearance of a TBI biomarker would be invaluable as a tool in determining when a player may return to full contact activity or when it is safe to return a soldier to the battlefield. Proteomic research in this field is ongoing in attempts to identify novel biomarkers in the cerebral spinal fluid that correlate with the severity of TBI and predictors of recovery.

Metabolomics

Metabolomics refers to the characterization of the cellular, small-molecule metabolite pool that is present in biological systems. It provides an overview of the metabolic status and the biochemical processes occurring in a given set of conditions. The metabolites that are studied include sugars, amino acids, lipids, steroids and triglycerides. Currently, over 40,000 metabolite structures have been characterized in the Human Metabolome Database, a freely available electronic database that contains extensive information about thousands of small molecules in the human body (http://hmdb.ca). Metabolomics allows for the opportunity to identify biomarkers or biomarker changes in biological fluids related to an environmental stressor. One application of this technique is the analysis of the urinary metabolic profile of kidney transplant recipients when evaluating for acute or chronic cellular rejection. If one could identify a unique metabolite for this process, then patients could be treated for rejection without the need for biopsy. Another application is in the setting of heart failure whereby myocardial biopsy is not readily available but several metabolic changes are occurring. Identification of metabolic abnormalities in heart failure could lead to the application of metabolomics profiling in detecting those at risk and targeting therapy toward specific metabolic pathways [10].

One advantage of using metabolomics is that biomarkers from metabolomic profiling studies can be translated from preclinical studies to the clinical setting since many endogenous metabolites such as sugars, amino acids, and lipids are species-independent, whereas gene transcripts and proteins often show interspecies variation. However, one disadvantage is that, in contrast to the human genome, the human metabolome is not well characterized. There are close to 3000 endogenous metabolites that are present in the human body and only a subset has been identified, characterized, and archived in web-accessible databases. Metabolic profiling is in its early stages but should continue to grow, as technology improves and more metabolites are identified and characterized.

Conclusions

Translational research is a viable and rapidly expanding field of research that allows the surgeon to identify molecular signatures or novel biomarkers for a given disease process that he or she manages clinically. Surgeons have the unique ability to identify the critical challenges in patient management, ask the appropriate research questions, and bring those questions to the laboratory for testing. Technologies for genomics, proteomics, and metabolomics are available and constantly improving so that scientists can continue to unravel the relationships of molecular signatures and protein biomarkers with disease. The development of a successful translational research program requires collaboration with a group of clinicians and scientists with the skills to develop an effective methodological strategy. In addition, the team needs to have the technical expertise to carry out the high-throughput, biochemical and molecular studies and analyses that can be correlated with clinical outcomes. The surgeon scientist can be the leader of this collaborative team. The development of a robust translational research program is a viable and rewarding career path that can lead to success in academic surgery.

References

1. Gerber DE, Minna JD. ALK inhibition for non-small cell lung cancer: from discovery to therapy in record time. Cancer Cell. 2010;18:548–51.
2. Tusher VG, Tibshirani R, Chu G. Significance analysis of microarrays applied to the ionizing radiation response. Proc Natl Acad Sci U S A. 2001;98:5116–21.
3. Modena BD, Kurian SM, Gaber LW, Waalen J, Su AI, Gelbart T, et al. Gene expression in biopsies of acute rejection and interstitial fibrosis/tubular atrophy reveals highly shared mechanisms that correlate with worse long-term outcomes. Am J Transplant. 2016;16(7):1982–98.
4. Harring TR, Guiteau JJ, Nguyen NT, Cotton RT, Gingras MC, Wheeler DA, et al. Building a comprehensive genomic program for hepatocellular carcinoma. World J Surg. 2011;35:1746–50.
5. Dowell JA, Frost DC, Zhang J, Li L. Comparison of two-dimensional fractionation techniques for shotgun proteomics. Anal Chem. 2008;80:6715–23.
6. Nelson PR, O'Malley KA, Feezor RJ, Moldawer LL, Seeger JM. Genomic and proteomic determinants of lower extremity revascularization failure: rationale and study design. J Vasc Surg. 2007;45 Suppl A:A82–91.
7. Tweedle EM, Khattak I, Ang CW, Nedjadi T, Jenkins R, Park BK, et al. Low molecular weight heat shock protein HSP27 is a prognostic indicator in rectal cancer but not colon cancer. Gut. 2010;59:1501–10.
8. Ren F, Wu H, Lei Y, Zhang H, Liu R, Zhao Y, et al. Quantitative proteomics identification of phosphoglycerate mutase 1 as a novel therapeutic target in hepatocellular carcinoma. Mol Cancer. 2010;9:81.
9. Guo J, Ren Y, Hou G, Wen B, Xian F, Chen Z, et al. A comprehensive investigation towards the indicative proteins of bladder cancer in urine: from surveying cell secretomes to verifying urine proteins. J Proteome Res. 2016;15(7):2164–77.
10. Hunter WG, Kelly JP, McGarrah 3rd RW, Kraus WE, Shah SH. Metabolic dysfunction in heart failure: diagnostic, prognostic, and pathophysiologic insights from metabolomic profiling. Curr Heart Fail Rep. 2016;13:119–31.

Selected Reading

Beger RD, Sun J, Schnackenberg LK. Metabolomics approaches for discovering biomarkers of drug-induced hepatotoxicity and nephrotoxicity. Toxicol Appl Pharm. 2010;243:154–66.

Cobb JP, Mindrinos MN, Miller-Graziano C, et al. Application of genome-wide expression analysis to human health and disease. Proc Natl Acad Sci U S A. 2005;102(13):4801–6.

Hirschhorn JN, Lohmueller K, Byrne E, et al. A comprehensive review of genetic association studies. Genet Med. 2002;4(2):45–61.

Hocquette JF. Where are we in genomics? J Physiol Pharmacol. 2005;56(Supp 3):37–70.

McDunn JE, Chung P, Laramie JM, et al. Surgical research review: physiologic genomics. Surgery. 2006;139(2):133–9.

Chapter 10
How to Write and Revise a Manuscript for Peer Review Publication

Melina R. Kibbe

Introduction

Writing is often regarded as an unfavorable or difficult task, and is frequently left to the last minute out of dislike, lack of confidence, or lack of know-how. However, writing can be fun, and the fruits of your labor can have substantial benefits. The purpose of this chapter is to convey to the reader why it is important to write, especially in academia, and why it is important to learn how to write and revise manuscripts well. Specifically, this chapter will address: (1) how to get started writing, including where and when to write and how to choose the appropriate journal; (2) how to write a manuscript for peer-review publication; (3) the order in which to write the manuscript sections; (4) how to respond to reviewer comments and revise a manuscript; and (5) how to use good English language grammar and effective writing strategies. In summary, this chapter is designed to provide a framework for authors to write, submit, and revise a manuscript for peer-review publication while at the same time deconstructing manuscript writing so that it can be an enjoyable, non-daunting task.

Why Write

There are many reasons why it is important to write and write well in academic medicine. First, publication deficiency is the single greatest barrier to promotion and tenure. Publication of research, whether it is basic science, translational, clinical outcomes, health services, or education research, is the primary measure of academic

---

M.R. Kibbe, M.D., F.A.C.S., F.A.H.A.
Department of Surgery, University of North Carolina,
160 Dental Circle, Burnett-Womack Bldg, Chapel Hill, NC 27599-7050, USA

productivity. Second, writing is a way to convey novel concepts and ideas to the academic community at large and contribute to the collective knowledge. Third, publication provides both personal and institutional recognition. Fourth, many faculty members leave academia as a result of failure to publish. Thus, if you are interested in achieving and maintaining an academic position, and/or interested in conveying novel concepts and ideas to a larger audience, you must become proficient at writing.

Getting Started

Where and When to Write

For most individuals, finding time to write is difficult in today's busy technological age with increasing pressures for clinical productivity. However, to be successful, you must make writing a priority. While some believe that the first three Rules of academic writing are: (1) just do it, (2) just do it, and (3) just do it, this is more easily said than done. It is important to recognize your writing style. Some prefer to write in long, quiet blocks of time. Others prefer short, repeated sessions. After recognizing your writing style, it is important to block out the necessary time on your calendar to write. For productive writing time, it is recommended to have an environment free from distractions such as emails and phone calls. If you are one of those individuals who needs constant email contact to feel in touch, then try at least muting the volume on your computer so you are not disturbed every time you receive an email. But, best practice would be to close the email application all together. Last, setting writing deadlines and adhering to them is important for maintaining consistent productivity. Cheating on your self-imposed deadlines only hurts you and your academic prowess, as it often leads to rushing, cutting of corners, and potentially sloppy work.

The place you write is equally important. If you have a busy personal life or have children, writing at home can be very difficult. However, if you have an open door policy at work, writing in your office can also be difficult as you may encounter many interruptions from people stopping by to ask questions and chat. Depending on your circumstances, you should decide where the best place is for you to write. Some may prefer finding a quiet hidden spot in the library with their laptop, while others may decide that a corner booth in a coffee shop is ideal. Merely closing your office door may be a sufficient signal to others that private time is needed and that you should not be disturbed. Regardless, find what works best for you and adhere to it. Having discipline is half the battle.

Choosing the Journal

Before you begin to write, it is critical to determine who your audience is so that an appropriate journal can be chosen. First, decide if your topic is of general interest or for a specific audience. Second, establish if it is related to basic science, clinical outcomes or health services, or education research? Third, determine the length of your publication. Addressing these three questions will help to distill the number of suitable journals to a manageable number. Once you have narrowed the list of potential journals, you should become familiar with the impact factor of those journals to further refine which one to select. The impact factor is a number that is generated annually from an equation that reflects the average number of times publications from that journal are subsequently cited in other articles. A higher number can be translated to mean that publication of manuscripts in that journal is more likely to have an impact on the scientific community, and is thus an indicator of the relative importance of that journal within its field. Frequently, promotion and tenure committees, society membership committees, award committees, etc., will evaluate not only the number of publications on faculty curriculum vitae, but also the impact factor of the journals and the faculty member's H-index (an author-level metric that reflects both the number of publications and frequency with which they have been cited). Therefore, it is important to publish your manuscript in the highest impact factor journal that is relevant and suitable for your publication. Last, it is important to look at the actual articles published in the journal to confirm that the journal publishes articles similar to yours. Browse the table of contents. If there is any doubt, choose another journal.

Instructions to Authors

After allocating time to write, deciding the best location to write, and determining the most appropriate journal for submission, it is imperative to obtain the "Instructions to Authors" from that journal. This should be done BEFORE any writing is commenced. The "Instructions to Authors" will outline the specific requirements for that journal, and these can be quite variable. Instructions will detail the total character count, word count, or page length for the manuscript, total number of figures and tables allowed; and total character or word count for the abstract. The precise format for the abstract will be provided, and typically includes a background, methods, results, and conclusion sections. Yet, to demonstrate the wide variability, while the New England Journal of Medicine requires the abstract sections described above, the Journal of the American Medical Association (JAMA) requires the following sections: importance, objective, design, setting, and participants, interventions, main outcome measures, results, conclusion, and trial registration. Thus, it is critical to obtain these instructions before starting to write and adhere to these instructions given the variability among journals. Some journals will reject manuscripts without review if these instructions are not followed.

Another aspect of the "Instructions to Authors" that is important is the actual type-set format used to prepare the manuscript document. While the majority of journals still require the document to be double spaced with specific margins (typically 1-in.) and specific sections, some journals have adopted a single-spaced approach or even double column single-spaced approach. Most recently, some journals have even adopted a "Your Paper, Your Way" format, which allows authors to submit manuscripts in any format they want, knowing the format will save time in the long run. Journals also have requirements regarding the use of abbreviations and references. Last, each journal has specific format requirements for figures. Many journals require the images to be Joint Photographic Experts Group (JPEG) or Tagged Image File Format (TIFF) images, with specific requirements for image resolution if they are color (i.e., 600 dots per inch, dpi) versus black and white (i.e., 300 dpi), however some journals do allow images from PowerPoint files or as portable document format (pdf) images. Therefore, attention to these details will save time, energy, and frustration on your part, since submission using an incorrect format will ensure either automatic rejection or annoyance on the part of the reviewers, with the latter potentially leading to a less than favorable review.

Writing

Manuscript Writing Order

The key to writing a good manuscript is to **tell a story**! This is often best accomplished by writing the manuscript out of order from the journal's prescribed order for the sections as certain sections are more logical and easy to write first, while others are easier to write after the bulk of the manuscript has been written (Table 10.1). I recommend starting with the figures and tables, as the figures and tables should tell the whole story, as well as a good story. Story boards are a helpful way to get this process started. Use one 8 ½″ × 11″ white sheet of paper and quickly draw the layout of each figure or table on one piece of paper. If there are five figures and one table, you should have six pieces of paper. This process helps to organize the flow of the figures and tables within the manuscript and determine precisely what data will be included. The reader should be able to surmise the overall message of the manuscript from the figures and tables alone.

Table 10.1 Recommended order to write the manuscript sections

Order number	Section
1st	Figures and tables
2nd	Title page
3rd	Methods
4th	Results
5th	Figure legends
6th	Introduction
7th	Discussion
8th	Abstract
9th	Acknowledgments
10th	References

After the figures and tables are determined, create the title page, carefully including all of the information required by the journal. Be sure to include all middle initials of authors if they are used by the authors, as well as correct institution information. After the title page, the methods (or materials and methods) section should be written, as this is simple to do and a logical lead into the results section. Next, complete the results section and organize this section using subheadings. This should be simple to write with the figures and tables in hand. While on your mind, after preparing the results section, it is convenient to write the figure legends. The introduction, followed by discussion should be written next. After you have all the other sections written, the introduction and discussion sections are less daunting to write. The last section to write is the abstract. A common mistake is to write the abstract first, before the results section. However, you will have a better sense of what to include in the abstract, as well as what to emphasize, after the majority of the paper is written. Remember, the abstract should include all pertinent data from the manuscript and accurately portray what is in the manuscript. Finally, don't forget the acknowledgements and references sections.

Figures and Tables

The figures and tables of a manuscript should **tell a story**. They should be clear to the reader without having to read or refer to the text of the manuscript. Figures should be necessary and relevant. Unusual aspects of figures or aspects of the data that need emphasis should be labeled with arrows or other indicators, drawing the readers' attention to these findings. Be careful and selective when including figures with negative data. While this can be very important to the overall message of certain manuscripts, more often than not, negative data are not sufficiently relevant to warrant a figure. Figures are used to emphasize data, and also to efficiently convey these data to the reader. For example, graphically depicting data with line graphs or bar charts may be easier than describing the data in the text. Tables are typically used to convey larger sets of data for multiple different treatment groups, allowing the reader to make comparisons between groups. Tables are also helpful when providing background information and experimental or clinical data, especially numerical data. Again, this is simpler than listing numerical data for multiple categories in different treatment groups in the text of the manuscript. A common mistake made by authors is to include data in a table or figure and also describe it in the text. This type of redundancy is unnecessary and will usually be detected by careful reviewers and editors. Not only is it annoying to the reader, but it takes up valuable print space in the journal, and that costs money. Therefore, it is best to limit your tables and figures to relevant data and avoid redundancy.

Methods

The methods section conveys to the reader what experiments or interventions were performed to address the hypothesis or question that was formed for the study. Methods should be described in enough detail so that the reader can judge whether the findings reported in the results section are reliable. Additionally, enough detail should be provided to allow the reader to reproduce the experiment. If the methods have been described in a previous publication, it is acceptable and advised to reference that publication and only briefly describe the methods. However, if deviations from the published methodology occurred, this should be clearly stated and described. If a new methodology is described, be sure to explain what experiments were conducted to test or validate the new methodology.

The methods section should be subdivided into descriptive subheadings. For example, the subheadings for a basic science research publication may include: cell culture, proliferation assay, western blot analysis, animal care and surgery, tissue processing, immunohistochemistry, and statistical analysis. For a clinical research study, subheadings may include: patient cohort, procedural details, subject follow-up, and statistical analysis. It is also important to indicate the purpose of why each experiment was performed in order to help the reader follow what was done. For example, the following indicates why a certain assay was performed: "To determine the effect of nitric oxide on the activity of the E2 enzyme, an activity assay was conducted using recombinant E1, E2, ubiquitin, ATP, and magnesium."

Results

The results section should **tell a story** and emphasize the take home message. The results section should state the results of the experiments and not contain conjecture. The latter is best left for the discussion section. Avoid repeating introductory material and minimize experimental details, since experimental details belong in the methods section. Avoid lengthy analyses and comparisons to other studies. Arrange the results section in a logical fashion, either chronologically, most-to-least important, *in vitro* to *in vivo*, etc. Organize the results section with descriptive subheadings. Here is an example of a non-descriptive and descriptive subheading: "eNOS Deficiency and Atherosclerosis" versus "eNOS Deficiency Increases Atherosclerosis." Remember the difference between data and results. Data are the facts obtained from the experiments and observations; results are statements that interpret these data. For each subheading section, I find it most helpful to state the purpose of the experiment(s) being performed to guide the reader seamlessly through these sections. After stating the purpose, the data are provided in a clear, concise, and logical manner. At the end of each subheading section, a statement is provided that summarizes and interprets the data, i.e., provides the results (e.g., "These data suggest that…"). This method is a very effective and efficient method to convey data and results to readers. The results section should also clearly direct the reader to the related figures and tables that support the data. Be sure to indicate, or "(see Table II)". In addition, it is important to avoid overlap between the text in the results section and the figures and tables. If data are described in a table or figure, there is no need to also list those data points in the text, as this is unnecessarily redundant. It is important to use descriptive sentence writing, and to display your experimental reasoning. An example of displaying experimental reasoning is: "To address this issue, we performed…." In summary, a well-laid out and well-written results section should be simple to read and should provide a clear story of the data for the reader to interpret and make independent assessments and judgments.

Figure Legends

After writing the results section, it is simple to prepare the figure legends, as these two sections are very similar. Use brief sentences to describe the figure. Different journals have unique requirements regarding the format. For example, some journals prefer including a title sentence for each figure legend that is description, while others do not. It is prudent to review publications from each journal to determine how figure legends are formatted. Figure legends should be free-standing from the text of the manuscript, meaning that a reader should be able to fully understand the experiment and data provided in the figure by reading just the figure legend, and not having to refer to the text of the manuscript. Describe all aspects of the figure, and if the figure has multiple panels, each panel must be described separately. Minimize experimental details, as that is the purpose of the methods section. All abbreviations, lines, bars, arrows, and symbols must be described. Provide statistical information; if the figure contains statistical notations such as asterisks, the P-values for these statistical notations should be provided in the figure legend.

Introduction

Grab the readers' attention with the introduction. Awaken the readers' interest and prepare them to understand the manuscript as well as its context to the scientific area being studied. Limit the introduction sections to three paragraphs and no more (Table 10.2). In the first paragraph, clearly state the clinical problem being addressed and its significance within the medical community. In the second paragraph, state what is known and then what is not known about the clinical problem. In the third paragraph, relate what is not known about the clinical problem to your study, providing clear support for why your study is important and being conducted. Then, clearly state the goals or aims of the study. Sometimes, the statement of purpose can be translated into a question; however, the more specific the better. Here is an example of a purpose posed as a question: "In this study, we asked whether an infusion of an cNOS inhibitor into the venous circulation will decrease hepatic arterial blood

Table 10.2 Content of the introduction section

Paragraph	Content
1st paragraph	State the clinical problem and the significance of the clinical problem within the medical community.
2nd paragraph	State what is known and what is not known about the clinical problem.
3rd paragraph	Relate what is not known to your study; clearly state the aims or goals of the study; clearly state the hypothesis.

flow." Finally, clearly state the hypothesis. An example is as follows: "Our hypothesis is that administration of an eNOS inhibitor into the venous circulation will decrease hepatic arterial blood flow." Make the introduction succinct; avoid a large number of citations. If the introduction is too long or confusing, the reader will lose interest and not read the rest of the manuscript.

Discussion

Many authors fear writing manuscripts because of the discussion section. However, if the discussion section is deconstructed to just five paragraphs, it can actually be fun to write, as most all discussion sections should be only five paragraphs in length and no longer. The discussion section is meant to answer or address the question or hypothesis that was posed in the introduction. It is also meant to relate findings and conclusions to existing knowledge. The discussion section should convey what exactly the study showed, what it meant, and how else it can be interpreted. Point out if other studies had similar results or disagreements and point out the study's strengths and weaknesses. Finally, convey what should happen next.

When writing the discussion section, several errors are common. First, do not restate the results. This is a crutch that many authors use if they do not know what else to put in the discussion section. Second, understate the conclusions rather than overstate them. Overstating conclusions is a certain way to annoy reviewers and readers. Third, be focused with your writing. Long, tangential thoughts make for sloppy and difficult to read discussion sections. Fourth, write clear and logical paragraphs with introductory and concluding sentences.

The discussion section can be written in five paragraphs (Table 10.3). In the first paragraph, summarize the results section and answer the question or hypothesis stated in the introduction. Place the data in the context of the bigger clinical problem. Examples of sentences that signal the answer include: "This study indicates that…", or "The results of this study show that…". Examples of sentences that link the results to the answer they support include: "In our experiments, we showed that…", or "In our subjects, we found that…", or "The evidence provided in this study shows that…".

The second and third paragraphs require the most thought and insight to write. First, use these two paragraphs to compare and contrast your data to existing literature. An example is: "Though our results may differ from those of Chen et al., we used a different method to ascertain compliance with therapy," or "While our results

Table 10.3 Content of the discussion section

Paragraph	Content
1st paragraph	Summary paragraph
2nd & 3rd paragraphs	Compare and contrast your study to published literature;
	Explain unexpected findings;
	Describe patterns, principles, and relationships with your results;
	Discuss theoretical or practical implications of the results
4th paragraph	Address weaknesses and limitations of the study
5th paragraph	Concluding paragraph

are opposite to those of Kao et al., we used a different rat strain with our studies." Second, explain unexpected findings. For example, "We were surprised to find that a normal WBC was predictive of morbidity following endovascular interventions." Third, describe patterns, principles, and relationships that the results show. Fourth, address if the results have theoretical or practical implications. Do the results relate to other situations or other species? Do the results help us to understand the broader topic? By addressing these issues, you will have provided the reader with additional insight into your study and how to place your results in context of the greater scientific field of study.

In the fourth paragraph, address limitations and/or weaknesses of the study. Let us be candid – there is no point in ignoring the limitations of your study. All studies have weaknesses and/or limitations and if you do not address them you are leaving yourself wide open for criticism by the reviewers. Thus, address the limitations and weaknesses openly and discuss why these limitations or weaknesses exist and how they may affect interpretation of the data.

The fifth and final paragraph should be the concluding paragraph. Provide a brief and global summary of the results and what it all means in context of the larger clinical problem discussed in the introduction. Signal the end using phrases such as, "In conclusion," or "In summary,". Indicate the importance of the work by stating the applications of the work, recommendations suggested from the work, implications of the work, or speculations about the importance of the work. Remember – do not overstate the conclusion – understate it.

Acknowledgments

The beauty of the acknowledgments section is its simplicity and importance. This is where most journals require the listing of support from funding agencies. Also, acknowledge individuals that contributed to the work but did not meet criteria for authorship. Gifts of special reagents, animals, software, etc. can be described here. Administrative support can be acknowledged. Of note, many journals now require that authorization be obtained from all individuals named in the acknowledgments section, so be sure to read the "Instructions to Authors" on this matter. Last, some journals ask for conflict of interest information or additional disclosure information in this section, or specifically have separate sections addressing those topics.

Abstract

The best time to write the abstract is after the manuscript is completed. The length of the abstract will be clearly stated by the journal and it is prudent to adhere to the length requirements. Sentence writing should be concise and succinct in the abstract, given the length requirements. Additionally, be careful to adhere to the formatting guidelines, as each journal has unique subheadings that must be used. In general, the abstract should provide an overview of the paper that makes sense when read alone AND when read with the paper. The abstract should provide enough information for the casual reader to understand what the manuscript is about. Include information from each section of the manuscript in the abstract, being careful to include, highlight, or emphasize important data and take-home messages, as often the abstract is the only part of the manuscript that is read. The abstract should not contain information that is not included in the manuscript. However, there may be some data in the manuscript that is not necessary to include in the abstract if it is not germane to the overall conclusion of the paper.

Title

A good title attracts the reader to the manuscript. Many readers scan tables of content or search engine results such as Pubmed. The title is typically the only aspect of the manuscript that can entice the reader to continue reading. The title identifies the main topic and/or message of the manuscript. A typical structure of a title is "The Effect of X on Y in Z," with the independent variable being X, the dependent variable being Y, and the animal or population or material being Z. It is wise to be precise with the title. Do not use "Effect of" when you mean "Proliferation of," or "Increase in," or "Reduction in". Last, be careful with the use of "and" and "with" when joining the independent and dependent variables. The following is an example of an ambiguous versus a precise title: "Arterial Diameter and Flow Rates in Porcine Arteries" versus "Arterial Diameter Determines Flow Rates in Porcine Arteries."

Authorship

Authorship is a very sensitive but incredibly important area. It is best addressed before the manuscript is written. Many journals have published guidelines indicating criteria that should be met in order to achieve authorship. In fact, many journals now require the corresponding author or each author to confirm that they have made a substantial contribution to the manuscript and indicate their precise role in the study. Each journal is different, but major areas for consideration include the authors' roles in (1) study design, (2) study execution/data acquisition, (3) data analysis, (4) manuscript preparation, (5) manuscript revision, and (6) final approval. Commensurate with these requirements, many journals now have a limit to the number of authors that can be included. If additional authors meet criteria for authorship that exceed the limit, most editors will allow an exception to the authorship number rule if the authors' roles can be documented. This is often done in the cover letter, or on the separate authorship role form, supplied by the journal.

The first author and senior author designations are traditionally the most important roles. The first author is usually the person who conducted the majority of the study and actually wrote the manuscript. The senior author is usually the person who provided overall supervision of the project, provided funding for the project, and has final approval on all aspects of the study and manuscript. In today's climate of multidisciplinary research, these designations are being challenged. Publications that represent work from several laboratories may have two investigators that truly contributed to the work equally and want to both receive first author status. In these situations, the first two authors can be listed with an asterisk on the cover page as sharing co-authorship. A common statement indicating this would be: "*H. Chen and L. Kao contributed equally to this work." Sharing senior authorship is an area that is also gaining popularity, I have personally adopted the use of "**M. Kibbe and G. Ameer share senior authorship" on my publications in which myself and my collaborator share funding and oversight of a project equally. First and senior authorship has significant implications for promotion and tenure. Thus, I hope that the Council of Editors will develop and adopt universal guidelines on how to address shared first and senior authorship in a manner similar to how the National Institutes of Health developed and adopted the multi-principal investigator mechanism for research grants. I also hope that promotion and tenure committees will recognize these designations and give appropriate credit for these designations when evaluating a candidate.

The last part of authorship that deserves mention is the use of the full name with the middle initial. In this electronic age, many investigators search Pubmed or Medline to find publications from a certain author. Use of the middle initial can help to distill the publications to only that author, especially when an author has a common last name. For example, search of Pubmed for "Smith M." revealed >14,000 publications. Search of Pubmed for "Smith M.M." revealed just over 400 publications. If Smith M.M. did not use his/her middle initial, it would be very difficult to locate all studies from that individual. Therefore, be consistent and try to use your middle initial on all publications.

Revising Before Submission

"There is no form of prose more difficult to understand and more tedious to read than the average scientific paper," according to Dr. Francis Crick in his 1994 book *The Astonishing Hypothesis* [1]. Learning to read and revise your writing is critical. In fact, "there is no such thing as good writing. There is only good rewriting," according to Harry Shaw [2]. Writing is simple. Re-writing is what makes a manuscript great AND fun to read. The ultimate goal of writing is to communicate your thoughts in a clear manner. Have the reader focus on your science, not wonder what on earth you were thinking when you wrote the manuscript. Make your manuscript easy to read. Often, it is helpful to have an independent person review and edit your writing. Write with your readers in mind. Choose words carefully and aim for precision. Use "increase" or "decrease" instead of "change", or use "rat" or "mouse" instead of "animal." Avoid wordiness, jargon, and word clusters. Use simple words such as "before" and not "prior to", or "after" and not "following." Use "apparently" instead of "it would thus appear that," or use "because" instead of "in light of the fact that." Do not use excessive or uncommon abbreviations. Abbreviations should be defined at first mention in the abstract and in the text, but should be defined only once. Do not use abbreviations if the word is only used twice. Avoid using abbreviations for science terms that are commonly associated with other meanings. For example, don't abbreviate neointimal hyperplasia as NIH, as most readers associate NIH with the National Institutes of Health.

For sentences, write simple declarative sentences and make clear comparisons. Do not compare apples to oranges. For example, write "These results were similar to the results of previous studies" instead of "These results were similar to previous studies." Avoid writing flaws by making sure the subject and verb make sense together. For example, use "Control experiments were performed" instead of "Controls were performed". Do not omit helping verbs. For example, "Cells were stimulated with each compound, and amount of NO production measured after 24 h" should be revised to "Cells were stimulated with each compound, and *the* amount of NO production was measured after 24 h." Last, write in the active voice, as use of the passive voice can make it difficult for the reader to understand what you mean. For example, the following construction uses the passive voice: "Why was the road crossed by the chicken?" Revising this sentence with the active voice results in the common saying, "Why did the chicken cross the road?" The chicken is the one performing the action, yet in the passive voice, the road was the subject. If English is not your first language, find someone who can help revise and correct the grammar of your manuscript.

For paragraphs, it is important to write structured paragraphs, and not have a free flow of ideas and multiple tangents. Make each paragraph about one main point. Paragraphs should have an introductory or topic sentence, supporting sentences, and a concluding sentence. Often, it is appropriate and helpful for the concluding sentence to be a linking or transition sentence to the next paragraph, connecting succeeding paragraphs. Keep paragraphs short, as the reader will get bored or annoyed. If a paragraph takes up an entire page, it can often be divided into two paragraphs based on the topics being discussed. Alternatively, watch out for paragraphs that are too short, as this can be seen as disjointed. Paragraphs with only two or three sentences are at risk of being of being too short.

Responding to Reviewer Comments

Have you ever fired off a quick response to an email and immediately regretted it? When you receive the comments from the reviewers of your manuscript, take a deep breath,… in,…and,…out,…and sit down. Read the comments. Then, put the comments away for a day or two. Do NOT start writing a response immediately. Responding to the comments immediately is one of the biggest mistakes authors make, as the comments may irritate the author and lead to responses that convey an angry tone. Being respectful to the reviewers is very important, since the revised manuscript and the response to the reviewer comments will most likely be sent back to the original reviewers. When drafting the Response to Reviewers document, respond to all comments and number them logically. It is considerate and preferred to copy and paste the reviewer's comment and respond to this comment indicating the response AND what changes have been made in the manuscript. Merely providing a response without providing the reviewer comments makes it hard for the reviewer to re-review a manuscript, as the reviewer would have to go back and forth between documents to determine which comment you are attempting to address. An example of a courteous response is:

> Reviewer #1:
> **1. The discussion could be expanded to discuss some of the discrepancies seen in the results rather than simply ignoring them. For example, is the effect of NO on upregulation of the proteasomal subunits a direct or indirect effect?**
> *Thank you for this suggestion. The discussion section has been expanded. We have now included a discussion postulating on the mechanism by which NO may increase protein expression. We have also included a paragraph discussing the possible significance of the different effects of NO on the trypsin-, chymotrypsin-, and caspase-like activities of the 26S proteasome.*

Responding to the comment without revising the manuscript accordingly is a fatal flaw. Remember, tone of the response is very important. Never argue with the reviewer. Modify the manuscript according to the suggestions of the reviewers as much as possible. If a reviewer asks for experiments beyond the scope of the manuscript, clearly state this in the response and address this in the cover letter to the editor. Additionally, if two reviewers are asking for opposing requests, choose which one to pursue and justify this in the response and point this out to the editor in the cover letter.

Conclusion

Writing can and should be an enjoyable experience. There is no greater ability than conveying to others new knowledge in the form of a good story. In addition, a career in academia is based on one's ability to publish. By following this simple outline on how to write a manuscript, and good use of English grammar and sentence structure, writing your manuscript should be simple and straight forward, and not the daunting task perceived by many. As said by a famous star ship captain, "make it so".

References

1. Crick F. The astonishing hypothesis: the scientific search for the soul. New York: Schribner; 1995. ISBN-10: 0684801582.
2. Shaw H. Errors in English and ways to correct them. 4th ed. HarperCollins Publishers New York, NY. ISBN-10: 0064610446.

Suggested Reading

Derish P, Eastwood S. A clarity clinic for surgical writing. J Surg Res. 2008;147(1):50–8.

Kane TS. The new oxford guide to writing. New York: Oxford University Press; 1994. ISBN-10: 0195090594.

Kibbe MR. How to write a paper. ANZ J Surg. 2013;83(1–2):90–2.

Kibbe MR, Sarr MG, Livingston EH, Freischlag JA, Lillemoe KD, McFadden DW. The art and science of publishing: reflections from editors of surgery journals. J Surg Res. 2014;186(1):7–15.

Strunk Jr W, White EB. The elements of style. 4th ed. Longman Publishers, New York, NY; 1999. ISBN-10: 0205313426.

Zeiger M. Essentials of writing biomedical research papers. New York: McGraw-Hill; 1999. ISBN-10: 0071345442.

Part III
Critical Elements for Success

Chapter 11
Choosing, and Being, a Good Mentor

Tracy S. Wang and Julie Ann Sosa

Introduction

Mentoring is considered to be an essential duty of academic surgeons. It is a catalyst for success in academic medicine, as mentoring relationships can facilitate career selection, advancement, and productivity among mentees. Unfortunately, there are important barriers to successful mentoring, such as increased clinical, research, administrative, and teaching demands on academic surgeons, along with the perception that mentorship is undervalued (or not recognized or rewarded) by many academic institutions. Is mentorship, then, an art that is in jeopardy of extinction?

In 2006, a systematic review by Sambunjak et al. of 42 articles describing 39 studies about mentorship in academic medicine demonstrated a relative paucity of strong evidence about the development of mentorship; however, it did yield several important findings [1]. Most important, "mentorship was reported to have an important influence on personal development, career guidance, career choice, and research productivity, including publication and grant success." However, less than 50 % of medical students and in some fields less than 20 % of faculty members had a mentor. In addition, women appeared to have more difficulty than male colleagues finding mentors. In one single-institution survey of medical students, residents, fellows, and junior faculty, 22 % of women junior faculty and 21 % of women residents had

---

T.S. Wang, M.D., M.P.H., F.A.C.S. (✉)
Division of Surgical Oncology, Section of Endocrine Surgery, Medical College of Wisconsin, 9200 W. Wisconsin Avenue, Milwaukee, WI 53226, USA

J.A. Sosa, M.A., M.D., F.A.C.S.
Section of Endocrine Surgery, Surgical Center for Outcomes Research (SCORES),
Endocrine Neoplasia Diseases Group, Duke Cancer Institute and Duke Clinical Research Institute, Duke University, DUMC #2945, Durham, NC 27710, USA

never had a professional mentor; in contrast, for men, the same was true for 9 % of junior faculty and 17 % of residents. In addition, men were three times more likely to describe a relationship with a mentor that positively influenced their career [2]. A more recent study of NIH K-award recipients from 2006 to 2009 demonstrated overall career satisfaction was related to the nature of a mentoring relationship and positive mentor behaviors. However, women were more likely than men to report having difficulty developing a relationship with a mentor (21 % vs. 18 %; $p<0.01$) and were less likely to identify someone whose career could serve as a model for their own (55 % vs. 40 %; $p<0.001$) [3].

A recent survey of National Institutes of Health (NIH)-funded members of the American Pediatric Surgical Association identified mentorship as one of the most important factors in their scientific success; however, in a 2004 study of women pediatric surgeons, 16 % of survey respondents reported that they never had a mentor [4, 5]. In a 2001 study, Thakur et al. found that 40 % of graduates of the University of California at Los Angeles general surgery residency program identified mentor guidance as important in personal development, and 38 % in research development [6]. Ko et al. in 1998 reported that 56 % of senior surgeons were influenced by a mentor in their choice of specialty, while Lukish and Cruess found that nearly half of surgery residents reported that mentorship played an important role in their decision to pursue surgical training [7, 8].

In the end, studies have shown that faculty members who identify a mentor feel more confident than their peers, are more likely to have a productive research career, and report greater career satisfaction.

Origins of the Term

Mentorship is a concept that dates from Greek antiquity. In Homer's "Odyssey," Mentor, son of Alcumus and friend of Odysseus, served as an overseer of Odysseus' son, Telemachus, and of his palace while Odysseus was away fighting in the Trojan War. When Odysseus did not return from the war, Athena, the goddess of wisdom, appeared in the form of Mentor to Telemachus, encouraging him to defy the suitors of his mother Penelope and go abroad in search of his father. It is interesting that some scholars argue that Mentor was ineffective, and that it was Athena, when disguised as Mentor, who provided the critical guidance that Telemachus needed in a time of crisis. This underlines the point that a good mentor can be an elusive entity, and mentoring often involves multiple individuals. Because of Athena aka Mentor's near-paternal relationship with Telemachus, over time the term 'mentor' in English has become synonymous with a father-like teacher, trusted advisor, friend, or wise person.

A more contemporary re-introduction of the term was in 1699 by the French author Francois Fenelon in the book Les "Aventures de Telemaque," which was intended to describe the educational travels of Telemachus and his tutor, Mentor, by summarizing many of Mentor's speeches and advice on how to rule [9].

Modern Definition and Primer

Today, mentoring is best described as a series of complex interactions between two individuals who have as their primary purpose the growth of the mentee, although this process often results in the personal and professional growth of both parties. Mentoring can involve a transfer of knowledge, patterns of behavior, skills, and an approach to an accumulated body of information. It sets the stage for mentees to approach, define, and mold their future and develop networks of peers, co-investigators, and colleagues.

Generally, a mentor is a more experienced person who can take several forms. Mentoring, as described by the National Academies of Sciences, Engineering and Medicine consensus statement on mentoring, is a personal and professional 'dyadic' relationship between a more experienced or senior person (mentor) and a less experienced or junior person (mentee). Informal mentoring occurs serendipitously when two individuals are drawn together by mutual interests and appeal, resulting in a kind of "spontaneous or accidental mentoring [that] almost always works." This type of mentoring is characterized by a long-term, mutually satisfying relationship that is not initiated, managed, or structured by an institution or organization. Hallmarks of the relationship are support, mutual respect, and compatibility. It is characterized by institutional proximity and by primarily direct, face to face contact. This generally excludes support from a distant site provided mostly through electronic media ("e-mentoring," or "virtual mentoring"), which, although similar to peer support in that it can be used for teaching, supervising, and counseling, can rarely by itself provide mentoring functions related to navigating the unique institutional environment and advocating for the mentee. It should be used as an adjunct, rather than a substitute, for an in-person relationship in order to maintain established bonds over time, particularly when the mentor/mentee moves or changes institutions, or when serendipitous associations are formed at national or international venues such as meetings or study sections. Mentoring is not synonymous with peer support, tutoring, teaching, coaching, supervising, advising, counseling, sponsoring, role-modeling, or preceptoring.

The traditional functions of the mentor have been viewed as almost exclusively supportive, such as writing letters of recommendation, assisting with publications, writing grants, and preparing for key negotiations. In this way, the ability to mentor does not necessarily require a position of power, but is often related to professional credibility. However, a mentor may also act as an advocate for the mentee; this type of mentor is often referred to as a 'sponsor'. Sponsorship has been defined as 'the public support by a powerful, influential person for the advancement and promotion of an individual within whom he or she sees untapped or unappreciated leadership talent of potential' [10]. The mentor/sponsor should promote the mentee in the department and the academic community at large, while at the same time protecting the mentee from the sometimes harsh interactions of academic surgery. Networking is an important and complex aspect of the mentoring experience that requires action by both the mentor and the mentee. The mentor can help the mentee gain access to otherwise 'closed' but important academic circles, and they should be willing to share their network of contacts and resources. Mentors can teach mentees how to promote themselves, as well as the 'rules of the game' of academic politics and networking. In the end, the effective mentor sets the stage for success by recognizing the potential of the mentee. The mentor must know the mentee well enough to envision possibilities.

A mentor is called upon to advise, advocate for, sponsor, and, when appropriate, constructively criticize the mentee in order to advance the mentee's interests and/or career. For mentorship to work, there must be a relationship or state of connectedness that is built on mutual trust and respect, as well as some personal chemistry; it generally develops over an extended period of time. As a result, it is the product of intense commitment and effort on the part of both the mentee and the mentor, and can come closer to a parent–child relationship than a teacher-student association. Mentees need to remember that most mentoring relationships are with a more senior faculty member and can result in a power differential where the mentee may be vulnerable. A recent survey of faculty members at two academic health centers found that five key features of a successful mentoring relationship were reciprocity, mutual respect, clear expectations, personal connection, and shared values (Table 11.1) [11].

In order for a mentee to choose the 'right' mentor, it is essential for the mentee to first understand what is needed and expected from the mentor to afford success. Insight comes from introspection. For example, is the mentee optimistic or pessimistic, and does the mentee respond to a more gentle or tough approach with regard to feedback and guidance? The mentee should be up front with a mentor about personal strengths and weaknesses, and about personal and professional goals: expectations should be clarified. To make the right choice of mentor, it is useful for mentees to 'interview' potential mentors as part of the selection process in order to find the optimal working, communication, and relational style. It may even be necessary to experiment with several different potential mentors in order to find the right match.

Some academic departments of surgery provide a formal mentorship program and 'designate' a faculty mentor for incoming interns, fellows, and junior faculty members; others suggest the creation of a contract between the mentor and mentee. Institutions should make women and minority mentors available to faculty members, but not assume that all mentees would prefer a mentor who is of the same gender or race. Most mentors in the National Faculty Survey of 3,013 full-time faculty in academic medicine were white men, a fact that likely highlights the limited numbers of women and minorities in senior positions in academic medicine [12]. Ideally, potential mentors and mentees would meet in social as well as professional settings to begin the networking process. This can serve as a starting point, but it should not be limiting. If a mentoring relationship set up by an institution feels forced or artificial, it is essential to acknowledge the problem. The mentee almost always should take the initiative of seeking out potential mentors, and patience and perseverance are required.

The best mentors are people who are excited about learning and who are continuing their own development, regardless of whether they are junior or senior academic

Table 11.1 Themes and illustrative quotes that characterize successful mentoring relationships from a qualitative study on successful and failed mentoring relationships through the Departments of Medicine at the University of Toronto Faculty of Medicine and the University of California, San Francisco, School of Medicine, 2010

Theme	Illustrative quotes
Reciprocity: bidirectional nature of mentoring, including consideration of strategies to make the relationship sustainable and mutually rewarding	Mentoring can't be something that is added to [the mentors] schedule and they have nothing to gain. I think that they have to perceive that they are gaining something from that relationship as well.
	It's got to be a two-way street. It can't just be a one-way giving relationship 'cause then it's just going to burn out. I mean I think the mentor gets a lot out of just the satisfaction of seeing their mentee succeed and that is important unto itself, that's the most important part but you know beyond that the mentor also needs some sort of tangible reward from the relationship that will kind of refresh them and make them keep wanting to come back for more. And that can be, you know, being on a publication or being recognized.
Mutual respect: respect for the mentor and the mentee's time, effort, and qualifications	Both individuals need to respect the qualifications of the other and the needs of the other and work together towards a common goal
Clear expectations: expectations of the relationship are outlined at the onset and revisited over time; both mentor and mentee are held accountable to these expectations	It's helpful to set up sort of those guidelines in the beginning, sort of what the mentee can expect from the relationship but also what the mentor expects you know, like "if you're working with me and you're going to be working on my data, you should publishing something off it" or "we're going to be working on grant proposals together" or that kind of thing
	Mutual accountability that the mentor has expectations of the mentee but the mentee also has expectations of the mentor
Personal connection: connection between the mentor and mentee	Mentors and mentees should have the "same chemistry" but not just being friends.
	There are many people that I did meet that had similar interests as me but there just wasn't a personal connection.
	Having that connection where you feel like someone actually cares to know what you're thinking and who you are and is really actually doing it because they care rather than because they're, you know, forced to
Shared values: around the mentor and mentee's approach to research, clinical work, and personal life	Mentorship worked when mentors and mentees were on a fairly common ground, have similar ideas and interests and values

Reprinted with permission from Straus et al. [11]

surgeons. They should be respected, and demonstrate good interpersonal skills and judgment. Good mentors actively participate in others' learning and growth. They also encourage and motivate mentees to move beyond their comfort zone to independence. In so doing, they achieve a sense of personal satisfaction from seeing others succeed. In this way, they are selfless. Mentees should seek out potential mentors who set high standards for their own work, thereby setting a real-life working example for their mentee(s). Finally, it is imperative to be honest with a potential mentor about why you want or need a mentor, and why you have selected him/her. Mentors should be willing to make a significant time commitment to the process, and both parties must keep the content of all communication confidential.

Overall, it is best if a mentor has an area of relative expertise that at least overlaps with that of their mentee, but it does not have to be an exact fit. For example, it is possible to have multiple mentors who complement each other with regard to the skill sets they can offer mentees; in particular, it is not uncommon for mentees to have different mentors for their research and clinical development, or for their local or national/international advancement. In addition, it is possible to have a professional career mentor and another mentor who offers advice about life outside of surgery. The down side of having more than one mentor is that it may mean having many different opinions about the appropriate course of action, leaving the mentee to sort through all of the disparate opinions before reaching a final decision about course of action.

A common tradeoff that must be made is between the time commitment that can be offered to counseling by the mentor and the academic rank or seniority of the mentor. Assistant and Associate professors tend to have fewer competing commitments and therefore more time to spend with mentees, but this comes at the expense of less experience and real-life wisdom acquired from rising through the ranks of academic surgery. The opposite is true among full professors and local and national leaders in academic surgery. Regardless of whether a junior or senior surgeon is selected to be a mentor, it is essential that an over-committed person not be chosen. Mentors who cancel meetings with their mentees or who are out of town, in the operating room or meetings, or simply unavailable in person, by phone and/or email are unlikely to make good sounding boards or counselors, particularly in times of crisis, since these are often unexpected and demand rapid counsel. Intermediaries, such as laboratory directors or administrative assistants, should not then become surrogates.

One way to predict accurately who is more likely to make a good mentor is to examine a mentor-candidate's track record of training or mentorship. As part of the promotion process at most academic institutions, it is common practice for academic surgeons to keep a record of medical students, graduate students, postdoctoral or clinical fellows, residents, and more junior faculty to whom they have served as an advisor or mentor; it is important to tease out the level of involvement the mentor had in the careers of each of the people on this list.

To do this, it is reasonable to ask a mentor to see their training record, and to examine that record for surgeon-scientists. It is also appropriate to contact former mentees' and ask them (in confidence) about their experiences. Finally, it can be useful to examine the mentor's publication list to see who serves as first author and senior author on peer-reviewed manuscripts. The best mentors propel their mentees' careers by placing them in the position of first author, while taking the senior author position.

Transition from Mentee to Colleague

While both advisors and mentors provide advice and guidance, mentors maintain a much higher state of connectedness with their mentees, and over a longer period of time. Indeed, many successful associations last a lifetime. Mentoring changes over time. If it is functional, a mentoring relationship develops over different phases, depending on the needs and resources of both sides. At some point, mentor and mentee may separate and redefine their relationship; otherwise, mentoring can become dysfunctional. It is critical that mentoring be a no-fault relationship that either party has the option to terminate for good reason at any time without risk or harm to careers.

There is no set time limit to mentoring. At some point, the relationship undergoes a transition as mentees seek guidance less often, and mentors gain a level of comfort with their mentees moving forward independently. Ideally, mentees and mentors establish a somewhat different relationship as colleagues, working together on projects of mutual interest. During the transition from being mentored to becoming colleagues, the period of increased independence needed by the mentee may create a sense of struggle; this can be disruptive to the relationship if the mentor does not truly support this. Open communication is tremendously important in this regard. It is also incumbent upon mentors to feel secure enough in their role, accept and embrace their mentee's growing independence, and celebrate their transition to colleague, as this is the best metric for the performance of mentoring.

Mentoring Risks

It is generally flattering to be called someone's mentor, and having a mentoring program for residents, fellows, and junior faculty usually increases the reputation of an institution. However, there are inherent risks to the mentee and to the mentor, particular in formal mentoring programs. Mentees may have unrealistic expectations, make unreasonable demands of their mentors, or may be unreceptive to mentoring altogether. When formal mentoring programs prescribe mentoring relationships, senior faculty can feel pressured into becoming mentors; as a result, they may be disinterested and unhelpful to the mentee(s) assigned to them. Within the inherent context of mentoring lies the potential for mentors to choose the easiest path and perpetuate the status quo or foster over-dependency, thereby failing to recognize and address the mentee's career goals, personal values, and needs. Finally, potential conflicts of interest should be avoided, especially if the mentor is in the position of being the mentee's direct supervisor. Mentorship should not aim for the mentee to evolve into a "clone" of the mentor; rather, it should foster a flexible environment that allows for the development of the mentee's own professional identity.

While it can be challenging to identify a good or even great mentor, it is equally (and perhaps more) critical to be able to recognize and avoid a bad mentor. Senior faculty who are hypercritical are often so because they are unable to share the limelight with mentees. Even subconscious jealousy may lead to a mentor's inaccessibility, desertion, or exploitation of the mentee. This can be exemplified by a mentor who usurps a mentee's work, pressures a disinterested mentee to continue involvement in the mentor's research, or inappropriately demands authorship. As mentees succeed in their own right and rise in stature and importance, it is conceivable that they will be perceived to be competitors, particularly because they share the expertise of their mentor. If mentors feel vulnerable or are insecure in their own right, they might fail (intentionally or unintentionally) to acknowledge the intellectual contributions of their mentees. This can result in acts of 'commission' or 'omission' that are not in the best interest of the mentee and can be perceived as being akin to bullying. Good mentors do not take credit or take over for their mentees; rather, they should celebrate their mentees' success, and convey that pride to the mentee and the community.

Finally, mentorship should never allow for even the perception of inappropriate personal boundaries; sometimes friendship alone can cloud judgment, and critical oversight is lost. Individuals may also experience unwanted romantic interest, sexual innuendo or harassment, coercive or other inappropriate behavior. If this is perceived, it should be addressed immediately. If the relationship cannot be repaired, it needs to be terminated in a safe environment for the mentee. When it becomes clear that a mentoring relationship is dysfunctional or non-productive, a mentee may want to involve a senior individual (e.g., the chair of the department or another very well-established, respected individual) before having face-to-face discussions with the mentor. Non-confrontational, open, and candid discussions can be uncomfortable, but they are very important. If the relationship is to be severed, it should be done expeditiously. It is extremely important that acrimonious or contentious issues not be perpetuated or discussed with others.

Conclusion

The most important metric of successful mentoring is the success of the mentee. The crucial issue is that mentoring, like all relationships, requires a significant time investment; if mentors do not have time and resources to devote, there can be no mentoring relationship. There are also benefits for mentors from mentoring junior faculty. These include developing a personal support network, information and feedback from their mentees, satisfaction from helping others, recognition (including accelerated promotion), and improved career satisfaction. Mentoring can, and should be, a reciprocally beneficial relationship.

In the end, mentoring has been shown to promote career development and satisfaction by increasing interest in one's career and enhancing faculty productivity, since it is linked to funding and publications. It also has been shown to facilitate promotion in academia, improve success of women and underrepresented minorities, increase the time that clinician-educators spend in scholarly activities, and perhaps even lead to less work-family conflict.

Acknowledgement The authors would like to thank Drs. Herbert Chen, Charles Scoggins, and Jennifer Tseng, all of whom provided their lecture materials from the Association of Academic Surgery Fall Courses for the creation of this manuscript.

References

1. Sambunkak D, Straus SE, Marusic A. Mentoring in academic medicine: a systematic review. JAMA. 2006;196(16):1103–15.
2. Osborn EH, Ernster VL, Martin JB. Women's attitudes toward careers in academic medicine at the University of California, San Francisco. Acad Med. 1992;67:59–62.
3. DeCastro R, Griffith KA, Ubel PA, Stewart A, Jagsi R. Mentoring and the career satisfaction of male and female academic medical faculty. Acad Med. 2014;89:301–11.
4. Watson C, King A, Mitra S, et al. What does it take to be a successful pediatric surgeon-scientist? J Pediatr Surg. 2015;50(6):1049–52.
5. Canaino DA, Sonnino RE, Paolo AM. Keys to career satisfaction: insights from a survey of women pediatric surgeons. J Pediatr Surg. 2004;39:984–90.
6. Thakur A, Fedorka P, Ko C, Buchmiller-Crair TL, Atkinson JB, Fonkalsrud EW. Impact of mentor guidance in surgical career selection. J Pediatr Surg. 2001;36:1802–4.
7. Ko CY, Whang EE, Karamanoukian R, Longmire WP, McFadden DW. What is the best method of surgical training? A report of America's leading senior surgeons. Arch Surg. 1998;133:900–5.
8. Lukish J, Cruess D. Executive Committee of the Resident and Associate Society of the American College of Surgeons. Personal satisfaction and mentorship are critical factors for today's resident surgeons to seek surgical training. Am Surg. 2005;71:971–4.
9. Fenelon, F. The adventures of Telemachus, the son of Ulysses. Edited by LA Chilton and OM Brack Jr. Athens: University of Georgia Press, 1997.
10. Travis EL, Doty L, Helitzer DL. Sponsorship: a path to the academic medicine C-suite for women faculty? Acad Med. 2013;88(10):1414–7.
11. Straus SE, Johnson MO, Marquez C, Feldman MD. Characteristics of successful and failed mentoring relationships; a qualitative study across two academic health centers. Acad Med. 2013;88(1):82–9.
12. Palepu A, Friedman R, Barnett R, et al. Junior faculty members' mentoring relationships and their professional development in U.S. medical schools. Acad Med. 1998;73:318–22.

Chapter 12
Writing a Grant/Obtaining Funding

Aaron J. Dawes and Melinda Maggard-Gibbons

Introduction: Can Surgeons Be Grant Writers?

Mentored Career Development Award Grants (also known as "K awards") are the portals through which the majority of academic investigators take their first step into the world of NIH-funded research. Compared with Research Project Grants ("R awards"), K awards are designed to provide aspiring researchers with a period of structured, protected, and mentored time to build their research skills and portfolio. This protected time and mentorship early in one's career matters--particularly for young academic surgeons with a busy clinical practice. An internal review of the K award program found that award recipients were significantly more likely than matched controls to apply for subsequent NIH grants, to be accepted for R awards, and to remain in research careers over the next decade [1]. While this career boost applied to K award recipients in general, it was most profound for M.D. and M.D./Ph.D. recipients, suggesting that clinicians may benefit disproportionately from this unique opportunity to focus on their own career development.

Whether due to the labor-intensive nature of their clinical work or a lack of experience in applying for grants, many young academic surgeons fail to take advantage of this important and accessible funding mechanism. Over the 15 years covered by the NIH's internal review (1990–2005), surgeons made up only 7 % of applicants for K08 awards and 2 % of applicants for K23 awards despite accounting for roughly 9 % of the faculty at academic medical centers. At least part of this disparity is due to lower application rates among surgical faculty: a 2004 study by Rangel and Moss found that surgeons were 2.5 times less likely than non-surgeons to apply for any

A.J. Dawes, M.D., Ph.D. (✉) • M. Maggard-Gibbons, M.D., M.S.H.S.
Department of Surgery, David Geffen School of Medicine at UCLA,
Los Angeles, CA, USA

type of NIH Career Development Award [2]. With stagnant or diminishing research budgets becoming the norm, it behooves young surgeons contemplating academic careers to become well versed in submitting successful grant proposals and developing the skills necessary to become an independent researcher.

Most of the information presented in this chapter is made freely available by the NIH on its various websites. However, these websites often bury valuable hints and tips beneath pages of technical information that require considerable time to both navigate and decipher. This chapter is an attempt to provide the applicant--especially the first-time applicant--with practical information for developing a well-crafted K award application. In particular, we describe what to look for in a mentor, how to write an innovative but feasible research plan, and how to avoid common errors in the application process.

While we designed this chapter as a guide to the application process, it does not attempt to summarize the full gamut of award mechanisms offered by the NIH. Furthermore, many of the principles outlined in this chapter can be applied to awards offered by other extramural funding agencies. Suffice it to say that the applicant's choice of award mechanism should fit with his or her career expectations and research plans. For example, clinicians pursuing laboratory-based research may find that the Mentored Clinical Scientist Research Career Development Award (K08) is best suited to their career goals while clinicians interested in research with more direct patient contact may gravitate toward the Mentored Patient-Oriented Research Career Development Award (K23). Your mentor can help guide you toward specific award mechanisms and should be integrally involved in the final selection. Even before talking to your mentor, applicants should spend time reading the guidelines and instructions for various awards on the NIH website (www.nih.gov). Communicating with the program officer at the appropriate NIH institute can also prove to be a valuable tool for learning more about a particular award mechanism.

There is no single formula for drafting a successful K award. There are, however, a series of concepts and tips that can maximize the likelihood of success. We have chosen to break the application process (and our guide) into four main sections: (1) understanding what the NIH is looking for in K award applications, (2) selecting an appropriate faculty mentor, (3) writing a successful award application, and (4) avoiding common pitfalls during the process. We hope that after reviewing this material young surgeons interested in an academic career will be better-equipped to develop stronger and more attractive K award applications.

What Does the NIH Want in a K Award Application?

Central to any application process is having a solid understanding about what the sponsoring organization and its reviewers are looking for--both in terms of the candidate and his or her research plan. Although the overall vision of these two groups should align, it is informative to separate what the organization wants from what its reviewers want to be sure that applications address both equally.

Perhaps the easiest way to determine what a NIH institute is looking for is by reading its mission statement, which can be found through the NIH website. Most share a general focus on understanding and treating human disease, in parallel to the NIH's own mission statement. But a closer reading can suggest areas of focus or even potential research programs. For example, the National Heart, Lung, and Blood Institute's (NHLBI) mission statement reads:

> The NHLBI provides global leadership for a research, training, and education program to promote the prevention and treatment of heart, lung, and blood diseases and enhance the health of all individuals so that they can live longer and more fulfilling lives. The NHLBI stimulates basic discoveries about the causes of disease, enables the translation of basic discoveries into clinical practice, fosters training and mentoring of emerging scientists and physicians, and communicates research advances to the public [3].

On a practical level, the first sentence of NHLBI's mission statement carefully lays out the institute's organizational chart and research divisions: Cardiovascular Sciences ("heart"), Lung Diseases ("lung"), and Blood Diseases and Resources ("blood diseases"). Any application to NHLBI that does not fit into one of these categories is at risk for rejection. Perhaps more importantly, the second sentence suggests fields of research that are of particular interest to the institute. In addition to basic science, NHLBI appears to be signaling an interest in both clinical translation and patient education, efforts that may align with its Center for Translation Research and Implementation Science and its Office of Science Policy, Engagement, Education, and Communication, respectively. All sponsoring organizations, including the NIH, are looking to fund projects that promote their underlying mission and goals. Applicants should take advantage of this by choosing an institute with goals that match their own and by describing their research plan in terms that align directly with the chosen institute's funding priorities.

Applicants should also keep in mind their reviewers, who may focus more on the practical issues of reading and scoring applications rather than on their Institute's long-term research goals. Successful applications pique reviewers interest, but they also demonstrate an awareness of their limitations. Although K awards are designed as stepping stones toward a future career in research, they must still produce tangible results and answer the questions they were designed to explore. For example, it is unlikely that a single K award will result in a cure for colon cancer. A reviewer faced with such a proposal may question the applicant's understanding of the science and his or her ability to perform the research within the funding period. Small, seemingly inconsequential errors in the application itself (even spelling) are often taken by reviewers as signs that the applicant lacks the skills, attention to detail, or mentorship necessary to accomplish the project. While some reviewers may be looking for the next big idea that will fundamentally change the field, others may simply be looking for easy ways to eliminate the 60–75% of applications that will not end up being funded [4]. Double-check everything with your mentor before submitting it. Do not give reviewers a reason to reject your application before fully considering it.

This focus on practicality and feasibility is not to say that successful applications steer clear of fundamental and important research questions. On the contrary: applicants must still convince reviewers that their work will change clinical practice or improve patient care, but a successful approach can be to break these larger questions into smaller, more feasible sub-questions that can reasonably be answered during the award period. *This balance between ambition and feasibility is among the most difficult, but most important lessons in writing a successful grant application.*

Selecting an Appropriate Research Mentor

Of the twelve tips on writing a successful K award provided by the NIH, six directly address the importance of the mentor (including the first three) [5]. In fact, many view the choice of mentor as the most important decision facing young faculty members and one of the most important determinants of K award success [6, 7]. Applicants should decide on their mentor long before drafting any components of the proposal. A common misconception is that K award proposals should be conceived of entirely by the applicant as a solo tour de force from beginning to end. Although the application should be independently written, reviewers expect mentors to be intimately involved throughout the process, including advising on important research questions, facilitating research collaborations, helping to outline experimental designs, critiquing rough drafts, and so on. The following comments may help in the selection process.

Select a primary mentor who is prominent and widely respected in your field of study. Someone with a substantial track record of NIH funding--preferably a R01 grant--is advantageous, but not essential. *A familiarity with the application process and a history of carrying out successful independent research, however, are considered prerequisites.* Your mentor should also be able to help you build and demonstrate institutional commitment for your application. This is especially important for surgeons looking to protect 50 % or more of their time for research. Either your primary mentor or an institutional administrator with control over your time and salary needs to emphasize their support for your application in their letter. Be sure to instruct whoever writes your letter of support not to imply that your academic position or faculty appointment is contingent upon receiving a K award; doing so may lessen the institutional commitment in the eyes of the reviewers.

Select a primary mentor who is either at your institution or close enough geographically to allow for frequent face-to-face meetings. Reviewers often scrutinize the frequency of these meetings when evaluating candidates, with weekly meetings being the norm. In addition to your primary mentor, your team should consist of one or more secondary mentors, each with a specific skillset that is essential to the success of your research plan [8]. For example, candidates who are new to surgical oncology and may have developed a relationship with a primary mentor outside of the field should consider including a secondary mentor who is an expert in the particular malignancy being studied. Your entire mentoring team should meet in person at least once every 2 months, if at all possible. If, for some reason, your research team is not in the same geographic location, you should plan to participate in conference calls or even web-based sessions as often as possible in order to avoid falling off track. Candidates should accentuate the importance of these virtual meetings in their application in order to convince reviewers that they will receive adequate support.

Select a primary mentor that you can work well with. It is often helpful to consider both the professional and personal attributes of your mentor and to reflect upon what type of mentoring relationship you typically thrive under. The National Academy of Sciences describes the mentoring relationship as a partnership, but stresses the mentor's role as an adviser, teacher, role model, friend, and advocate [9]. Some applicants will want a more "hands-on" approach to the mentoring relationship in which the mentor is available to outline and review initial materials. Others will prefer more freedom to struggle, make mistakes, and learn from those mistakes on their own. Whatever strategy you prefer, be sure it aligns with your mentor's style of teaching and his or her track record with junior faculty. You might even want to seek out your mentor's prior mentees to learn about their experience and to get some guidance on how to maximize the mentoring relationship. At the end of the day, your mentor's ability and willingness to communicate the lessons he or she has learned along the way will be key to your success during the award period and during your transition to research independence.

Experienced mentors will recognize the mentor letter as their main opportunity to influence reviewers. A well-written letter directly communicates the mentor's support for the project, but also implies that the mentor has set aside time to formulate a plan specific to the mentee, to write the letter, and to review and revise the research plan. Common subheadings include: (1) Candidate's Qualifications and Relationship with the Mentor, (2) Mentor's Qualifications, (3) Philosophy/Views on Mentoring and Mentoring Experience (including a table of previous trainees showing their training period, degree earned, research project, funded award, current position), (4) Why the Mentoring Team was Chosen and their Qualifications, (5) Nature and Extent of Supervision, (6) Mentor's Comments on Career Development Plan and Research Plan including Limitations of the Plan, (7) Measurable Milestones and Outcomes, (8) Timeline of Activities, (9) Institution's Mentoring Policy, and (10) Experience with previous K awardees. Although length does not substitute for substance, a detailed mentor letter is often interpreted by the reviewers as one of the best predictors of success, not only during the K award period, but also for the applicant's long-term pathway toward independence.

Finally, be sure that your primary mentor reviews your entire application prior to submitting it. Minor factual mistakes, scientific errors, and other technical flaws are all clues that the mentor did not thoroughly review your work. You may consider having another faculty member who is not on your mentoring team or even a faculty member outside of your field or institution read your application and critique it. For example, surgeons without a basic science background may benefit from enlisting a Ph.D. colleague to comment on their methods for handling and analyzing tissue samples. Identifying potential areas of weakness in your application before submitting it will prevent future difficulties--either during the review process or when you actually go to carry out your research.

Writing a Successful Award Application

After selecting an award mechanism, an institute, and a mentor, researchers must begin the formal application process by putting together their written application. Regardless of the amount of outside work you put into your project, your application will be the main direct connection between you and the funding source. As such, it is imperative that your application accurately summarizes your proposed research project and does so in a way that will excite reviewers. Remember, most institutes will ask both experts in your field of interest and accomplished researchers outside of your field to review your application [10]. Do not assume that reviewers will automatically grasp the importance or novelty of your work; be sure to put your work into a larger clinical context and demonstrate how it will enhance clinical care or future research on the topic.

All K award applications are graded on five separate criteria: the Candidate, the Career Development Plan, the Research Plan, the Mentor, and the Environment [11]. In addition, reviewers are asked to give a global score from 10 (Exceptional) to 90 (Poor) based on the overall impact of the work. This final summary score was specifically added to integrate the significance of the proposed work with the feasibility of the research plan. Given that most applicants will already be associated with an institution and a clinical department, we have chosen to focus on the first three criteria (Selecting an Appropriate Research Mentor was discussed in the previous section). Since more detailed information on each criterion is available on the NIH website [11], our goal here is to synthesize the most important components of each criterion and to provide practical advice on developing a successful written application.

The Candidate

Unlike other funding streams where the primary focus is on the research *plan* rather than the research *team*, Career Development Awards are designed to live up to their name. The main goal of K awards is to develop future researchers not necessarily future research. For that reason, **K awards are as much about the person and his or her future potential as a researcher as they are about the research that he or she has proposed**. Successful applicants must be able to clearly, thoroughly, and emphatically "sell" reviewers on their ability to become independent researchers after the grant period. Reviewers want to be convinced that they will read your name again on successful R awards and will be able to follow your future academic work through national meetings and peer-reviewed publications.

Several tips may help to convince reviewers of your research potential. First, tell a story that connects your prior experiences to your current goal of becoming an independent researcher. Detours along the way are acceptable and must be thoroughly explained to reviewers, but do your best to weave a cohesive and convincing narrative about why you decided to pursue an academic career and how your future research will improve upon and enhance your current clinical practice. A surgical narrative might sound like this:

> I chose a career in surgery to focus on treating patients with cancer, but during my clinical training I realized that removing pancreatic tumors after they have become symptomatic cannot substantially reduce the burden of disease. I now understand that only by exploring the scientific bases of this disease--specifically the molecular signaling of pre-cancerous pancreatic cells--can I hope to truly improve the care of my future patients. To do this properly, I have decided to pursue a career in laboratory-based research.

Focusing on past experiences that highlight your desire to pursue further scholarship can be helpful as well. Maybe you gave lectures to medical students and junior residents about the pathophysiology of pancreatic cancer. Maybe you worked to develop a registry for following cancer patients treated at your institution. If you are an M.D./Ph.D., be sure to comment on how your proposed research is related to the independent work you did for your Ph.D. Even summer internships as a medical student that demonstrate an innate desire to learn and improve that can help to paint the picture of you as a future scholar in the field.

Second, draw from your past experiences and from those of your mentor, but demonstrate a desire to work independently. Since surgery requires considerable clinical responsibilities that may compete with your time to perform research, it is especially imperative that surgeons effectively communicate their desire to pursue an academic, research-based career. Remember, reviewers are overworked and may skim your application before reading it in depth. It can be useful to repetitively re-state that your goal is to become an independent researcher.

Third, lean on prior publications, national/international presentations, or substantive preliminary data as a demonstration of your commitment to research and your growing expertise in your field of interest. More than a publication count, reviewers are looking for signs of productivity: does this applicant have the skills and commitment necessary for delivering real academic output? If your publication record is limited, be sure to mention other projects on which you have taken leadership roles, even if they have not yet led to publications (e.g., managing an ongoing clinical trial or helping to set up a research clinic in another country) [5]. It is a good idea to feature any peer-reviewed manuscripts you have written with your mentor because they help to demonstrate an established mentor-mentee relationship. At the same time, be sure to emphasize that the project you are proposing is distinct from your mentor's work. K awards are only designed to last 3–5 years; after that, awardees are expected to apply for more significant grants as a principle investigator. Applications should demonstrate an applicant's ability to build on previous work and to identify new topics or sub-fields of research that will become the basis for a long career in academia.

Fourth, ***address any potential limitations head on***. Do not dismiss as unimportant any educational gaps in your career. Clearly explain what happened, why your career progression was interrupted, and how you are now moving back on track. More damage is done by being silent in the hope that the reviewers will not notice the time taken off. In the same vein, a poor publication record is not necessarily seen as a prognostic sign of future academic failure. Again, clearly explain why this happened (e.g., inadequate mentorship or institutional support) and then explain how you will overcome this limitation in your Career Development Plan. If you need to resubmit a grant application, be sure to take the time in between submissions to publish at least one peer-reviewed manuscript with your mentor. Even a small clinical case report or a short review article that marginally relates to your proposed research can suffice. Your commitment to academic research and further evidence of a supportive and productive mentor-mentee relationship will be duly noted by the reviewers.

The Career Development Plan

By far, the most frequent error made by K award applicants is underappreciating the importance of an organized, fluidly written, and well-designed Career Development Plan. Remember, K awards are not just smaller R awards. While both offer a source of funding for research, ***K awards are also designed to provide junior faculty members with an opportunity to gain the experience and training that they will need to achieve independence by the end of the granting period***. The Career Development Plan is your opportunity to show *how* you plan to achieve this goal: what skills are you currently lacking, what areas do you need to develop, and what steps will you take to fill in these gaps in knowledge. It may help to organize your plan into short-term, mid-term, and long-term goals, but be sure to be specific about what you plan to do during the award period (typically the first 3–5 years). The Career Development Plan is also the first section that many reviewers read and, as in life, first impressions matter.

Several simple tips can help you produce an organized and customized Career Development Plan. First, take stock of your academic deficiencies, both in terms of the research outlined in your award application and your future career. The best award proposals develop an educational program that is unique to the applicant's research interests and technical needs. Maybe your research involves the importance of diet on colon cancer risk, but you have never formally studied nutrition. In this case, you might propose a plan that includes graduate level courses in dietetics. Similarly, you may have earned a Ph.D. in cell biology, but may have no background in biostatistics. You might use your award period to pursue a degree--or a series of courses--in statistics to demonstrate that you will have the tools you need to complete your proposed analyses. In an R award, applicants typically supplement their lack of knowledge in a particular area by relying on a consultant or colleague with that particular expertise. Although reviewers for a K award will still expect you to have a mentor with an appropriate knowledge of the subject matter, a larger emphasis is placed on the applicant becoming an expert in his or her proposed field of study.

When considering a formal degree program, be sure that the degree (and the time committed to formal coursework) fits within your larger Career Development Plan. Certain degree programs, such as a Masters of Public Health or a Masters of Science in Clinical Investigation, incorporate many courses that are critical to the development of any young investigator, such as basic statistics, epidemiology, and bioethics. On-line courses should generally be avoided since it is difficult for the reviewers to judge their quality. Courses should not be spread thinly across the award period; instead, try to finish them in the first 2 or 3 years so that the remaining time can be devoted to research. A table or figure with course names, objectives, and degree requirements can make the reviewers' job easier. Timelines should be detailed and specific so that reviewers can tell exactly when you plan to complete your didactic work. Remember, it *is* possible to take too many courses. Most applicants will have already spent nearly a decade in postdoctoral training learning to be a surgeon; the goal now is to fill in any remaining gaps in knowledge before embarking on your future academic career.

Second, every junior faculty member must face the balance between clinical work and research. There is no easy answer to how and where to spend your time. As a surgeon with ongoing clinical responsibilities and a need to maintain the operative skills developed during training, it may be hard initially to find time to commit to research. This balance should be discussed with your primary mentor, co-mentor, or institutional representative before submitting your application. Reviewers typically want a detailed description of your planned clinical responsibilities during the award period, including how many cases you plan on performing each week, what your call schedule will be like, and what kinds of additional support you will have to deal with clinical issues that arise during your non-clinical days. It may also be helpful to specify the hours per week you expect to spend in class or on homework during the beginning of your award period. It is critical that your mentor also addresses all of these topics in his or her letter of support. As with every part of the award application, clarity and feasibility are key. Reviewers need to understand how you plan to maintain this balance and need to be convinced that you will have the appropriate support to carry out your plan.

Third, be sure that the information coming from you and your mentor align perfectly. Review your Career Development Plan with your mentor before submitting. Ask for his or her input and be sure what you have written closely matches what the two of you have discussed. Lack of communication between mentor and mentee or inconsistencies between the goals and objectives each has set out are a harbinger of a failed mentor-mentee relationship--and a serious red flag to reviewers. Your mentor's letter should lay out the milestones you will need to meet in order to achieve promotion (i.e., papers to be published, national presentations to be given) and your Career Development Plan should clearly state how the award will propel you towards each of these milestones. If you have already established a relationship with your primary mentor--maybe you are co-authors on a manuscript, textbook chapter, or similar publication--be sure to emphasize this in your Career Development Plan. Demonstrating a stable working relationship is important, but be sure to lay out for reviewers how you will build upon this prior relationship in your future work.

Research Plan

Although the Research Plan is often the most straightforward portion of the application, it can also be among the most difficult to write clearly. Before you write anything, take some time to develop a strategy for your research. Start by performing a literature review or by talking to other faculty members who have done work in your field of interest. What are the major topics or areas of research that have generated interest over the past couple of years? Do any of them align with your interests or skill set? After you generate an initial list of potential research ideas, be sure to check out similar grant applications that have already been funded by the NIH [12]. Reviewing previously funded grants can prevent you from duplicating someone else's research and can help you hone in on the type of work that individual Institutes are interested in at this point in time. Grants can be reviewed online through the NIH's Research Portfolio Online Reporting Tools (RePORT) system (available at report.nih.gov). Applicants should also be aware of and try to play to the strengths of their home institution. Reviewers often discuss why a candidate did not utilize the available resources, especially if his or her university has been designated a "Center of Excellence" in a particular area.

Four key points should be kept in mind when drafting your Research Plan. First, try to highlight the importance and uniqueness of research. To borrow an idea from venture capital, applicants must generate a sense of "FoMO" in their reviewers--*a "Fear of Missing Out" on the chance to support the next big thing, the next great idea that will change the face of healthcare* [13]. Successful applications don't just present novel methods or test previously unexplored hypotheses; they tie the science back to curing, treating, or preventing disease [12]. If your work will help elucidate the intra-cellular components of a trans-membrane signaling protein, be sure to discuss how that information can be used to develop targets for new medications or improve the way we understand or treat a certain disease. If your work involves developing a new method for measuring patient satisfaction, comment on how your method could be used to make care more patient-centered or to track patients' recovery after surgery. Do not expect reviewers to automatically grasp the importance of your work. It is your job to convince them that your application should be selected from the pile of qualified submissions and the best way to do that is to demonstrate the potential downstream impact of your work.

When presenting preliminary data to support your proposal, be sure to consider their validity and be forthright about their source. Do not try to impress reviewers by passing off others' data (including your mentor's) as your own; almost invariably the result will be the exact opposite. Reviewers are surprisingly adept at knowing and finding out what your mentors are doing. If databases or websites are used in your preliminary data, how reliable are these sources? Have they been validated? In what setting? For example, if you are citing the results of a particular survey, have those data been replicated? Have they been replicated in a population similar to the one you are interested in? If not, these steps may need to be included at the beginning of your Specific Aims.

Second, while every effort must be made to stress the downstream impact of your research, ***proposals must be feasible given the applicant's skills, resources, mentorship, and timeline***. If you have no experience in statistics, be careful proposing a large secondary data analysis without adequate assistance from your research team. If you are studying a specific gene mutation's effect on chronic pancreatitis, be sure you are using the appropriate animal model. Asking another faculty member who is in your field, but is not one of your mentors to review your proposal may be helpful here. Some investigators may even be willing to share a copy of their own funded projects with you so that you can see what it takes to be successful [14]. An outside set of eyes--especially one with an expertise in the area in which you plan to work--can often catch small logical fallacies or inaccuracies that you may have missed.

As we have stressed throughout this chapter, remember that you are submitting a Career Development Award and not a R01 grant. While your end goal may be to find a cure for thyroid cancer or to redesign the Medicare system, it is unlikely that you will do so during your award period. Research Plans that are too narrow may fail to capture the interest of reviewers, but Plans that are too broad also present potential red flags. Reviewers may begin to question your understanding of the science or of the Award mechanism itself. Maintaining a proper balance between innovation and practicality is essential to writing a successful K award application.

Third, communicate your ideas clearly and succinctly. This is often best accomplished by focusing your proposal into no more than three Specific Aims and then organizing the remaining sections of your Research Plan directly around these Aims. Although they are physically separated in the grant, the Specific Aims section and the Research Plan should be thought of as one continuous entity. Background and preliminary data should be condensed so that your Specific Aims fit on a single page and reviewers should be able to understand the nuts and bolts of your project by reading this page alone. Again, balance is important when selecting your Aims. While you should not make the mistake of subdividing your three Specific Aims into four or five sub-aims, you also need to be sure that each Aim is substantial enough to stand up on its own. Many reviewers worry that, if Specific Aim 2 seems to be reliant on the completion of Specific Aim 1 and Specific Aim 1 fails, then the entire project will be irreparably damaged. Be careful not to propose three particularly time-consuming Specific Aims, like three randomized multicenter clinical trials. Reviewers want to be sure you will have the time to not only engage in mentored research, but to pursue other types of scholarly activities that will enable you to eventually take the next step into independent research.

Fourth, choose an appropriate study design and justify your choice. For example, you may decide that a prospective cohort design is more appropriate than a randomized clinical trial. If so, be sure you know and comment on the inherent biases to both designs and how your choice might impact your anticipated results. Here, assistance from your mentor and from other supporting faculty members is key. Beyond discussing your design at the outset of the application process, be sure to allocate the necessary time for your mentor to read (and re-read) your methods section and to comment extensively on your drafts before submission. Research plans that are not reviewed by mentors are obvious to reviewers and reflect poorly on both the applicant and the mentoring team. A knowledgeable mentor, for example, is often skilled at including critical references. Experts on some study sections will immediately recognize when important references have been overlooked and judge accordingly.

Especially if you are proposing clinical, translational, or health services research, consulting a statistician early on in the design process may help you avoid common methodologic or analytical errors. A statistician can help you perform sample size calculations, advise you on your patient accrual goals, pair down overly optimistic effect sizes, and, most importantly, tighten the writing in statistical sections. This can be particularly helpful since many review committees have a statistical reviewer who can often sense after reading one or two sentences if the candidate has consulted with a statistician or not. If you are performing a clinical trial, pay close attention to your recruitment and retention details. Do you have a plan to use a patient navigator for non-English-speaking patients or a study coordinator who can speak the requisite foreign language? Ensure that you have an appropriate control arm for all clinical studies and remember to include a data monitoring plan for any project involving an intervention, even a behavioral one.

Although you will be using more scientific language, you should think of your method section as telling a narrative, namely how you will move from planning to data collection to the generation of results, including what alternative approaches you plan to employ if problems arise. A generalized version might sound like this: "In my initial work, I discovered X. Now I plan to do Y and Z. If the result is A, then I will do B; but if the result is C, then, instead, I will do D." Be thorough--especially with respect to your plan for negative results--but keep your narrative simplistic. A useful strategy is often to pretend that you are explaining your research to a 10-year-old: "I am trying to kill cancer cells with a new medication, but if this doesn't work, I am going to try adding a different medication to see if the two medications work together to kill the cancer cells."

In addition to the content of your work, it is worth paying attention to several important organizational and formatting tips. Everything that reviewers need to consider your application should be included in your submission. Reviewers should not need to refer to any supplementary material to understand the background or significance of the research. If your study is nested in a larger application, provide the essential details of the larger grant, such as characteristics of the sample population and data collection methods, and be sure to distinguish your Specific Aims from those of the parent grant. Towards the end of the Research Plan, include a section on its limitations. These may include threats to either internal or external validity that you plan to control for with your approach. For example, a survey that is administered only in English may not produce findings that apply to non-English-speaking populations and, while similar, the pathophysiology of pancreatic adenocarcinoma in a mouse model may not perfectly match what is seen in human disease. Italicize and embolden important points or phrases to make them stand out to reviewers who may spent less time looking at your application. Limit the use of acronyms. They may be more convenient for you, but they often make the proposal harder to read and may confuse reviewers. Remember that the appendix has no space restrictions.

Use it to your advantage by adding details that may help reviewers understand your work, but are too lengthy to include in the text, such as outlines, validated questionnaires, or complex statistical plan. Beware, however, that not all reviewers read the appendix thoroughly, so all essential documentation needs to be provided in the main application.

Writing a well-thought-out and clearly constructed application is time consuming. Be sure to start the application process months in advance and aim to have a complete draft at least 1 month before the official due date. This is usually the bare minimum your mentoring team will need to review and comment. As with aspects of clinical surgery, careful planning and appropriate preparation can often obviate the need for last minute panic and help you put your best foot forward.

Conclusion: Top Ten Common Mistakes to Avoid

Even applicants who understand what the NIH wants, select an appropriate mentor, and produce a clear and innovative research plan can be tripped up by small, seemingly-inconsequential mistakes. Luckily, many of these mistakes are common--especially among first-time applicants--and can be avoided, if you know what to look out for. As a summary of our earlier sections, we conclude with our "top ten" common mistakes to avoid along with several simple tips on how to avoid them.

1. *Focusing more attention on the Research Plan than on the Career Development Plan*. As we mentioned throughout the chapter, K awards are unique in their focus on developing the applicant, not just his or her research. Applicants who submit a well-thought-out Research Plan, but a hastily compiled Career Development Plan may be surprised to find their application denied. The best Career Development Plans are organized, thorough, and, most importantly, tailored to the applicant's weaknesses and research needs. Take an honest look at your current skill set and your future career plans and then describe *in detail* how the time and resources of a K award will help you develop into an independent researcher.
2. *Selecting an inexperienced mentor or one that is too far outside the field of interest*. K awards are not just aimed at "career development"; they are meant to support "mentored career development," which means that your mentor needs to play a central role in both the application and the subsequent research activities. Ideal mentors have been through the process before and can help you overcome challenges and maximize your academic output. Before selecting a mentor, be sure that he or she offers you the subject-level expertise you will need, is available and willing to help, and has a plan for what to do if and when your project hits a standstill.
3. *Developing a Research Plan that cannot be accomplished during the award period*. Remember to balance innovation with feasibility. Your K award should be a first step toward research independence, not your life-long research plan.

4. ***Including a Career Development Plan that lacks sufficient detail regarding the training that will occur during the award period.*** Be explicit. Use a table with course names and numbers if you are planning a formal degree. And be sure to account for all of your time--clinically, in research, and on formal and informal educational activities.
5. ***Selecting team members or collaborators that are not based at the applicant's institution or not describing how the applicant will receive guidance remotely.*** Selecting an offsite mentor is a risk, but one that can pay off if the person you select offers you exactly what you need to be successful. If you do choose an offsite mentor, remember that reviewers may question your decision for fear that you will not receive adequate support; it is your job to convince them otherwise.
6. ***Not providing letters of support for all research team members or institutional representatives.*** Reviewers will undoubtedly question why these are not included with your application. Does the applicant actually know the people on his or her mentoring team? Will the institution actually support the applicant if the award is granted? Or did the applicant simply forget to include the necessary paperwork? Remember, failing to follow directions is always a red flag to reviewers.
7. ***Not working closely enough or early enough with institutional grant officers.*** Grant officers exist to help applicants through the application process. Use them. Do not wait to have your application rejected before learning that you have failed to meet a particular deadline or to fill out a necessary application form.
8. ***Not following the specific instructions for the grant application components.*** Instructions, while occasionally painful, are there for a reason. Read them and re-read them before submitting. If you have any questions at all, contact the program officer.
9. ***Not providing enough details on the applicant's clinical responsibilities.*** Reviewers want to be sure that you will have sufficient protected time to work on your research and to participate in your planned career development activities. Do not leave out information about your clinical responsibilities in the hope that reviewers will overlook your busy schedule; applicants are best served by being open and honest about their time commitments, especially surgeons, whose clinical work is often less predictable.
10. ***Demonstrating poor "grantsmanship" in the written application*** (e.g., submitting dense text without the use of figures or tables, not identifying and correcting spelling or typos, etc.). Although grants are not awarded based on prior NIH experience, reviewers can tell that someone is submitting for the first time if his or her application looks different from what has become standard among grant writers. Use the format to your advantage and make it seem like you have been there before, even if you haven't. Looking at other faculty members' grant applications and having a seasoned grant writer review your application prior to submission can go a long way in terms of giving reviewers exactly what they are looking for.

In contrast to conventional wisdom, the long clinical experience and unique perspectives of even junior level surgical faculty enable them to be fierce competitors for NIH Career Development Awards. It is incumbent on the young academic surgeon to seek the proper mentorship, craft an individualized course of didactic study, and work together with his or her mentor to develop an innovative yet feasible research plan. With the help of a well-disciplined approach, surgeons can write and win these coveted awards and go on to become excellent, independent scientists that contribute significantly to our understanding of human disease.

Acknowledgements Malcolm V. Brock for his work on an earlier version of this chapter.

References

1. National Institutes of Health. National Institutes of Health Individual Mentored Career Development Awards Program. US Department of Health and Human Services; 2011. https://grants.nih.gov/training/K_Awards_Evaluation_FinalReport_20110901.pdf.
2. Rangel SJ, Moss RL. Recent trends in the funding and utilization of NIH career development awards by surgical faculty. Surgery. 2004;136(2):232–9. doi:10.1016/j.surg.2004.04.025.
3. National Institutes of Health. The NHLBI mission statement. nhlbi.nih.gov. https://www.nhlbi.nih.gov/about/org/mission. Published August 2014. Accessed 20 Jan 2016.
4. National Institutes of Health. Research Portfolio Online Reporting Tools (RePORT): Table #204, NIH Career Development (K) Grants. report.nih.gov.
5. National Institutes of Health. Advice on Mentored Career Development Awards. niaid.nih.gov. http://www.niaid.nih.gov/researchfunding/traincareer/pages/mentorK.aspx#e1. Published January 31, 2012. Accessed 20 Jan 2016.
6. McDonagh KT. Identifying grant funding: mentored career development and transition awards. Hematology Am Soc Hematol Educ Program. 2008;2008(1):12–5. doi:10.1182/asheducation-2008.1.12.
7. Pollock RE, Balch CM. The NIH clinician-investigator award: how to write a training grant application. J Surg Res. 1989;46(1):1–3.
8. Morris AM. Funding sources in faculty development: strategies for success in submitting proposals. Clin Colon Rectal Surg. 2013;26(4):224–7. doi:10.1055/s-0033-1356721.
9. Committee on Science, Engineering, and Public Policy, National Academy of Sciences, National Academy of Engineering, Institute of Medicine. Adviser, teacher, role model, friend: on being a mentor to students in science and engineering. Washington, DC: National Academy Press; 1997. doi:10.17226/5789.
10. Milgram SL. NIH Grants 101: funding mechanism, peer review, and strategies for success. postdocs.stanford.edu. http://postdocs.stanford.edu/education/PDFs/NIH_GRANTS_STANFORD_FEB_2011.pdf. Published February 2011. Accessed 19 Jan 2016.
11. National Institutes of Health. Definitions of criteria and considerations for K critiques. grants.nih.gov. http://grants.nih.gov/grants/peer/critiques/k.htm. Published April 15, 2015. Accessed 29 June 2015.
12. Khachaturian H. Writing a successful career (K) application. 2011. http://www.fau.edu/research/nih/files/2011writing_career_app.ppt.
13. Kaplan K. Funding: got to get a grant. Nature. 2012;482(7385):429–31.
14. Wiseman JT, Alavi K, Milner RJ. Grant writing 101. Clin Colon Rectal Surg. 2013;26(4):228–31. doi:10.1055/s-0033-1356722.

Chapter 13
Setting Up a 'Lab' (Clinical or Basic Science Research Program) and Managing a Research Team

Fiemu E. Nwariaku

Introduction

As a brand new Assistant Professor, the surgeon-scientist is generally excited about starting a new job as well as the possibilities for building their very own research program. However, there is perhaps no greater source of anxiety for the young scientist than setting up and staffing a new research program (either in basic bench research or patient-oriented translational research). In this chapter, we provide very broad guidelines and advice to help avoid those pitfalls and build a successful research program. We also admit that there are numerous approaches to each of these elements and the recommended approaches delineated here, represent a fraction of available options. Although many of the references described in this chapter relate to bench research, the concepts can be applied broadly to any research program including clinical research programs. This chapter is deliberately written in a broad, informal and somewhat humorous style. The suggestions and recommendations are based on information distilled from multiple sources, while trying to be as practical as possible. As much as possible there are no references to specific techniques, research designs etc. At the end of the Chapter, there is a suggested reading list which contains useful material from which we have obtained some of this material. It is our hope that the new surgeon-scientist who is starting their scientific career will find this information useful in avoiding the most common pitfalls in setting up their research programs. We hope you enjoy it.

F.E. Nwariaku, M.D., F.A.C.S., F.W.A.C.S.
Malcolm O. Perry Professor of Surgery, Department of Surgery,
UT Southwestern Medical Center,
5323 Harry Hines Boulevard, Dallas, TX 75390, USA

In general most new surgeon-scientists bring tremendous energy to the new program. They possess a valuable skill set including a strong clinical background, awareness of scientific methods, and a strong personal motivation to succeed. However they usually need to learn new scientific methods, particularly in the basic sciences and establish new professional relationships while taking on an increasing clinical and teaching workload. All these factors are crucial to success but can also undermine productivity. As a result it is important to begin the process of setting up your research program deliberately, methodically and with the end product in mind.

Decisions, Decisions!

It can be overwhelming starting a new research program. The new scientist is often required to make major decisions for which many of us are poorly prepared. Decisions such as what kind of research personnel should I recruit and hire? How much should I pay them? How do I gauge their skill level? Should I share laboratory space with other investigators? How much should I spend on equipment? Unfortunately, many new investigators receive no formal training in laboratory or program design and organization because this is generally not taught in most training programs. However it is perhaps these may be most important tasks for the young surgeon-scientist. Furthermore poor program design can destroy the program and career of the investigator as well as the careers of other staff or trainees. It is also difficult to attract talented trainees and researchers to a poorly structured research environment. A few practical hints:

- Decide what values are important for you and your research program (e.g., scientific excellence, discipline, teamwork, competition)
- Develop a 5-year plan with the following questions:
    - What are my career goals?
    - Do I want to get tenure in 5 years?
    - Am I interested in entering a competitive research field?

Mission Impossible: Defining a Laboratory Mission or Vision

Of all the choices that an early stage investigator has to make, deciding what NOT to do may be the most difficult decision. New investigators usually have boundless energy and a wide spectrum of ideas without the scars of professional failure to temper their enthusiasm. As a result, a common mistake is to begin too many projects. A program mission becomes very important to provide focus for the investigator and the program in general. Like all important projects, creating the program mission should begin with the end result in focus. A program vision–either publicly displayed or stored in a private note book–is important to the success of your program. It is critical to formulate this plan **before** beginning the job search, for the following reasons:

- The vision determines which jobs and institutions that you will seriously consider (e.g.,. one would not look for a clinical research -intensive position in a university medical center with low clinical output).
- The vision facilitates a better understanding for the material and personnel needs for the job.
- This will also guide the negotiations for a start-up package

In the few weeks after accepting a position you should;

- Generate a prioritized list of resources and equipment needs.
- Obtain information from company vendors about discounts or start-up specials.
- Get an e-mail account at your new department and have your address added to group e-mail listings.
- Order reagents that do not require special storage.
- Meet with departmental financial and purchasing administrators.
- Meet with your immediate supervisor, Division Chief or Department Chair to discuss your ambitions and goals.
- Seek and establish collaborations within your institution!

Project Planning

Planning projects ensures that necessary resources are available prior to starting the project, and ensures that you seek and secure the resources that may not be available. A short check list should include the following:

- Create a resource list (Animals, human samples, radiation).
- Obtain institutional approval (IRB, IACUC).
- Compile a list of equipment and supplies and divide it into resources that are expensive and resources that are essential to your lab.
- Prioritize your spending needs.

Saving Money

Take the opportunity while visiting departments to ask about specific institutional resources: you can save tremendously by sharing instruments that are already in-house. Scientists are generally willing to give or share equipment when asked.

General lab supplies- tubes, glassware etc. will cost about $10,000 a year for each researcher. Other options are to buy generic electronics at electronic chain stores. These usually cost less than the institutional supply companies. If your institutional regulations and policies allow it, you can further save by purchasing equipment like refrigerators and microwaves at appliance stores.

Guide to your shopping list:

- Brainstorm.
- Come up with a number of ideas that you want to pursue as individual experiments.
- Rank your projects according to experiments that will yield preliminary data more quickly than others.
- Categorize the list.
- Check what equipment is available at your future department.

Purchasing

- Learn how to order supplies.
- Learn institutional and state regulations regarding purchasing (What is the approval process? how long does it take? Will it be delivered to the lab or to a central location and picked up by lab personnel?).
- Ask faculty and technicians in your department, and in others, if they have equipment they haven't used in a long time.
- Seek broken or very old equipment that can be fixed.
- Seek used and refurbished equipment vendors over the Internet.
- Look for the institutional salvage yard for desks, shelves, and file cabinets.
- Identify vendors that have contracts with your institution and ask your colleagues for the vendors that have the best sales representatives. This becomes particularly important when major equipment breaks down.
- Develop relationships with company representatives. They can be very helpful with discounts and specials. Some companies have a laboratory "start-up" program.

Seek Help

Take advantage of your current environment to ask colleagues for pointers and advice: ask how difficult (or easy) it has been for them to settle down into their labs; what were their biggest lab set-up problems? Another good idea is to include your email on departmental group e-mail lists.

People

Next to time, laboratory personnel represent the most important resource that we control. Our goal should be to hire the best personnel (match skill and experience with task complexity), that we can afford. Poor decision-making and lack of discipline when hiring laboratory personnel can truly destroy any chances of success. Furthermore many academic institutions require the employee (you), to provide significant amounts of documentation and due process when trying to terminate their employment. We have found the Human Resources (HR) department to be invaluable during recruitment, termination and everything in between. Some HR departments can also create a job description based on your laboratory needs, advertise the job and pre-screen potential candidates. Their expertise is invaluable; however they need to be contacted early during the process. It is strongly recommended that the scientist arrange to have meetings with the HR personnel within a few weeks of settling into his or her new position. During the meeting, discuss local hiring policies and practices. Obtain information about the institutional applicant pool. Examples of questions to ask include:

- What levels of employee are available within the institution?
- How skilled are they?
- Have they worked in large productive laboratories or programs?
- Are there any laboratories shutting down and do they have skilled personnel?
- What specific institutional guidelines exist for salary and benefits, insurance, incentives, duration of probationary employment, etc.?

Finally it is crucial to adhere to HR the policies and guidelines provided by your HR office, because failure to do so places your entire institution at significant legal risk!

Whom Should I Hire?

Generally most laboratories recruit four types of personnel: research technicians (also called research assistants or associates), postdoctoral fellows, graduate students, and undergraduate students. The first is considered research staff while the last three are trainees. Some scientists make the distinction between hiring staff, and recruiting trainees.

The nature of tasks to be performed generally dictates the type of personnel to be hired. It is helpful to first identify the necessary tasks for your projects. Specifically determine a reasonable time frame and grade the complexity of the experiments. Short-term, low complexity projects can be accomplished with a relatively new research technician or graduate student. Long term complex projects will require a more experienced research assistant/associate or a postdoctoral trainee with experience. It is important to remember that severe mismatching of personnel with projects can lead to poor productivity and frustration on both sides. However alignment of project and personnel can create job satisfaction, increase productivity and improve the work environment. Questions to ask during the hiring process include;

- What experimental methods or techniques will this individual be performing?
- How many years of experience should they have?

- Can I get the same expertise through a collaborator?
- Can I hire and train the individual?

The answers will provide your HR office with a sketch of the potential job description, which will in turn determine the salary range. Many HR offices can also assist with the interview process.

Advertising

It is important to advertise these positions broadly. Most institutions have websites maintained by the HR department where local and outside candidates routinely check for information. It is also helpful to cast a wide net by calling your colleagues in other institutions or posting the position on scientific websites. Some useful websites for advertising include;

Science (http://recruit.sciencemag.org),
Cell (http://www.cell.com),
Nature (http://www.nature.com),
Federation of American Societies for Experimental Biology's Career Resources, (http://career.faseb.org/careerweb/),
Science's Next Wave, (http://nextwave.sciencemag.org/jobsnet.dtl)
Association for Women in Science (http://www.awis.org/)

References

Always check at least two references from prior employers, colleagues or collaborators! We prefer a personal phone call or physical meeting, instead of email letters of reference, if possible. A personal phone call to the last employer is particularly important because many scientists are more comfortable providing honest feedback in person or on a phone call. The more referees you call, the more accurate your assessment. However one should avoid getting bogged down by numerous referee calls. Most people can get an accurate assessment after speaking to between 3 and 5 referees. Some guidelines for referee conversations include the following:

- Describe the job and the work atmosphere you want to create.
- Ask open-ended questions.
- Ask questions which require descriptive answers that are neither right nor wrong.

   Sample questions include:

- What was their greatest contribution during their time in the laboratory?
- Why is this person leaving?
- Is he or she reliable?

13 Setting Up a Research Program

- Would you rehire this person?
- What are this person's strengths and weaknesses?
- What are you most disappointed in with respect to this person?

Interviews

Conduct a Structured Interview

According to the book "Making the Right Moves: A Practical Guide to Scientific management for Postdocs and New Faculty", one should watch out for the following red flags during the interview process:

- Being unwilling to accept responsibility for a poor outcome.
- Complaining about previous supervisor, peer or subordinate.
- Demanding privileges not given to others.
- Delaying answering questions, challenging your questions, or avoiding answering them all together. (Humor and sarcasm can be tools to avoid answering questions.)
- Exhibiting anger or frustration during the interview,
- Acting incongruously from what they say (e.g., downcast eyes and slouching are not signs of an eager, assertive candidate).
- Trying to control the interview and otherwise behaving inappropriately.

Probation Period

Most institutions have a probation period during which you can terminate employment without a long process of documentation. Always confirm with the HR department when this period ends and be sure to address any performance deficiencies with the employee prior to the end of probation. Trainees are considered different and may not be subject to the same rules, however there are mechanisms to address performance issues with a trainee through the Student Office or the Postgraduate School.

Trainees

The primary role of the trainee in a research program is to learn. The concept is that during their trainee period, they will learn how to

- Ask important questions.
- Choose appropriate experimental methods designed to provide answers to those questions.
- Develop and hone their analytical skills to provide reasonable analysis of their observations.

- Develop skills to synthesize the often varying observations into a conclusion.
- Learn to communicate their ideas to peers, supervisors and the general scientific audience.

The last part involves learning presentation and grant writing skills as well as writing skills. It is OUR responsibility to ensure that these skills are developed. Therefore implicit in your decision to accept a student or postdoctoral fellow in your research program is the agreement to provide all the above training. This also requires significant time commitment to instruct, support, teach and supervise trainees. Because of this commitment, some scientists suggest that brand new investigators should refrain from taking students or trainees for several years after they start the laboratory. Also a bad experience for any trainee may not only turn them off science forever, but negatively impacts your ability to recruit bright and hardworking trainees in the future. Having said that, students are perhaps the most exciting to have in the laboratory. They are usually scientifically 'innocent'; they are eager to learn and often ask questions that lead down previously unexplored scientific paths. In general, undergraduate students enjoy learning basic experimental methods such as ELISA assays, microscopy and electrophoresis gels. These experiments allow them to fail and learn to solve technical problems without using up expensive reagents or jeopardizing valuable specimens.

In contrast, graduate students and postdoctoral fellows are usually more experienced and can attack more complex scientific problems with more sophisticated assays. A specific group of postdoctoral trainees is the clinical resident who takes time from their clinical training to learn about scientific research methods. Unlike the Ph.D -seeking postdoctoral fellows, many clinical residents often desire a robust publication record in a relatively short time. They may face stiff competition when they apply to clinical subspecialty fellowships, and the publication record improves their chances of securing admission. It is certainly prestigious to have a resident in the lab. However, we recommend that the surgeon-scientist be as objective as possible keeping the interest of the resident in the forefront of all discussions during this process. Several questions that need to be asked include;

- Is this the appropriate training for the resident?
- Is this the appropriate time for them to take the time to train?
- Are they committed to a lifelong career in scientific investigation or are they just curious?
- What is their clinical track record? In this instance, past activity is usually an indicator of future performance.
- Are their expectations realistic? Two to three publications each year (one laboratory and one or two clinical papers) is reasonable. Four to five good quality publications is difficult but outstanding if accomplished.

This group of trainees also has specific needs. Some of them may choose to engage in low level clinical activity such as moonlighting while in the lab, or they may take time to travel for interviews. Different groups address these issues differently. However, it is crucial for the surgeon-scientist to set clear expectations BEFORE the trainee is accepted. Most scientists understand that the primary reason for spending additional time training to become a clinician –scientist is so that they can learn the above mentioned methods. This requires a significant time and effort commitment. We discourage residents who do not grasp this concept from spending additional time in research training. A frequently asked question by trainees is the duration of their research training. Most training programs expect their residents to spend 1–2 years engaged in research. This decision can be made together with the trainee; however in our opinion, many projects that address important questions require at least 2 years to acquire the necessary information and publish it. Regardless of the skill level of trainees, it is important to remind ourselves that they all require instruction and mentoring.

Trainee Funding

Trainee funding can be a challenge for young scientists. However many major institutions have training grants in Departments that may not be the primary department of the investigator. We recommend that you contact the Office of Grants Management and get a list of training grants. Some clinical departments can also support the salary for trainees as part of their educational mission. However you will need to ask the Department Chair or Research Director. Lastly, many professional organizations such as the Association for Academic Surgery, Society of University Surgeons as well as specialty societies in vascular, colorectal, oncologic, cardiovascular and orthopedic surgery have established funding programs for student or postdoctoral trainees. Information on these programs can usually be found on the society websites. Regardless of the source of funding, the process needs to commence early. We recommend that trainees are identified and proposals submitted no later than a full year prior to the proposed start date. This allows the research programs enough time to prepare to receive the trainees, and also time to review research proposals and develop the research projects. It is crucial to communicate directly and clearly with the potential trainee and their residency program director during the entire process. It can be disheartening to prepare for a whole year to receive a trainee, and secure funding only to find out that the residency training program cannot afford to release the resident for the training period.

Time is (NOT) on Your Side

Many managers describe the concept that time is our most precious resource. Therefore it is crucial to learn, understand and practice great time management. Workshops and symposia about time management abound. Some institutions provide free workshops on time management to increase the efficiency of their employees. Take advantage of these, if your institution has one of these programs.

Whether we like it or not, academic productivity is judged by the number and quality of published papers and grants. Our product is discovery and new knowledge in the health sciences. Therefore our academic time should be spent on activities that facilitate increased production. Some writers discuss the investment of time. For example, spending time reading papers and rearranging your laboratory, may not directly lead to increased productivity, but time spent training staff on complex experiments can yield great returns in the future.

Research Techniques

A common pitfall early in one's career is the love affair with specific research techniques. Some investigators are enamored with a particular new technique. It is important to remember that research techniques are tools. Just like a hammer or screwdriver, each technique has advantages and weaknesses. Picking the right technique(s) for your project is very important. First, newer techniques are generally considered to be superior by reviewers. However some new techniques have not been adequately validated. Also, new techniques are generally more difficult and require a learning curve. As such the new investigator has to decide whether to (a) continue to use familiar techniques learned during training and maximize productivity or (b) develop a new technique to establish independence. This decision is guided by superiority of the new approach over the old, applicability of the new technique to the project, available resources, feasibility of the new approach, and cost.

Some new techniques are easily acquired, especially if it involves purchasing a new piece of equipment. Biomedical companies continue to strive to make measuring biological activity simpler, faster and more accurately. Unfortunately many of these machines come with a significantly large price tag. The price tag also includes service contracts and disposables. The new scientist should include all these costs in the calculation about whether to purchase the equipment. The patient-oriented researcher also has to deal with more powerful computing power, and expensive costs for detailed sophisticated biostatistical analysis. A relatively useful tactic is to use institutional core facilities when possible. Some cancer centers offer significant discounts to their members. It can also be helpful to teach in some basic science departments in return for discounts for use of core facilities. Examples of these facilities include molecular imaging, flow cytometry, confocal microscopy, tissue profiling cores and transgenic cores etc. Collaborating with colleagues who also serve as core Directors (if your research has the scientific basis and is similar) is also a good way of getting free core services. Negotiation is key.

Program Leadership

Leading a research effort is truly an immense privilege. The surgeon scientist has an opportunity to direct the search for new knowledge in a new field, share that information with the scientific community and shape young minds as they begin their own quest for scientific inquiry. This privilege comes with significant responsibilities. The Principal Investigator/Program Leader has similar responsibilities to the CEO of any company. They need to provide strategic direction for the research program, recruit and retain good personnel and put out a great product. A short list of responsibilities for the laboratory leader includes:

- Setting scientific direction
- Motivating personnel
- Communication
- Resolving conflict
- Mentoring
- Ensuring good academic output

Summary

In setting up a new research program, the new scientist has a tremendous opportunity to make important contributions to the health sciences and hopefully improve the lives and health of many people. Despite the numerous pitfalls, a methodical strategic plan, smart recruitment and creative budgeting can all greatly improve the chances of setting up a successful research enterprise. It is hoped that the contents of this chapter will assist in some small way and ease the transition from new scientist to established successful surgeon-scientist.

Bibliography

1. Harmening DM. Making the right moves: a practical guide to scientific management for postdocs and new faculty.
2. Harmening DM. At the helm: a laboratory navigator by Kathy Barker.
3. Harmening DM. Laboratory management: principles and processes. Upper Saddle River: Prentice Hall; 2003.

Part IV
Work-Life Balance

Chapter 14
Work-Life Balance and Burnout

Kathrin M. Troppmann and Christoph Troppmann

Introduction

Serious consideration of work-life balance and its impact on professional performance and family life have been anathema to generations of surgeons in training and in practice for much of the past century. William Halsted (1852–1922), the father of the first formal surgical residency training program in the United States at Johns Hopkins Hospital, demanded continuity of care from his residents. The restrictive lifestyle and extreme personal sacrifice that characterized Halsted's training program in the waning years of the nineteenth century remained pervasive in most American surgical training programs for much of the twentieth century—well into the 1960s and 1970s. During those earlier days, surgical residents frequently lived on hospital premises during their residencies, were strongly discouraged from starting families, and were not receiving salaries. Instead, they were gratified with room and board, hospital clothing, and with professional education and training. The Medicare and Medicaid Act of 1965, which was primarily designed to provide for medical care for the elderly and the poor, became one of the first agents of change in the surgical residents' lives in that it provided for a substantial salary [1]. The basic underpinnings of the surgical residency changed gradually, with surgical residents now at least physically spending part of their lives outside of their training institutions. It was not until the beginning of this new millennium, in the wake of the highly publicized Libby Zion case, that the Accreditation Council for Graduate Medical Education (ACGME) designed and mandated the 80-h workweek for surgical and other residents, placing, among other measures, a cap on the length of the shifts that could be worked [2]. Not surprisingly, this change regarding surgical residents' work hours generated vocal dissent from some of those representing prior

K.M. Troppmann, M.D., FACS • C. Troppmann, M.D., FACS (✉)
Department of Surgery, University of California, Davis School of Medicine, 2315 Stockton Blvd., Sacramento, CA 95817, USA

surgical generations. For instance, Josef Fischer, M.D. stated "The 80-h work week is seen as damaging to the essence of surgery's being. It is the denial of the foundation of...continuity of care." [3]

Nonetheless, the recognition of the importance of, and the focus on, work-life balance and related issues has continued to increase, fueled in part by the entry of Generation Y and the Millennials into the surgical workforce and by the increasing presence of women in the surgical workplace over the past decade and a half [4, 5].

This trend has been most strikingly evidenced by the appearance of peer-reviewed articles dedicated to surgeons' work-life balance, lifestyle issues, career satisfaction, and burnout, to name only a few issues. These articles have been published in steadily increasing numbers since the beginning of the new millennium in highly regarded scientific mainstream surgical journals [5–23]. This latest evolution has thus rendered the study, analysis and discussion of these topics completely acceptable—even for those academic and nonacademic practicing surgeons who may represent prior generations. In the future, it will be paramount, in light of the physician and surgeon shortage predicted for the coming decades, to direct appropriate attention to surgeons' lifestyle issues in order to ensure sufficient recruitment and retention of future generations of surgeons.

The purpose of this chapter is (i) to review the available evidence on work-life imbalance as experienced by currently practicing surgeons, (ii) to analyze the adverse consequences of work-life imbalance and burnout, and (iii) to describe potential strategies to address these issues at a personal and professional level.

Surgeons' Work-Life Imbalance and Its Consequences

Work-Life Imbalance: Magnitude of the Problem

There is ample evidence in the literature for a significant imbalance between work and life that is perceived by a substantial proportion of currently practicing surgeons.

In a recent national survey of surgeons (in all specialties and practice settings), 33 % reported that they did not achieve work-life balance [23]. This perception was independent of gender, age, marital status, presence (or absence) of children, academic or nonacademic clinical practice setting, surgical subspecialty and practice location (rural vs. urban). Fifty-nine percent of the queried surgeons believed that they worked too many hours and, of those, 59 % felt that the area most frequently affected by working too many hours was "family life" [23]. According to that survey, respondents spent an average of 20 h per week with family and friends and only 4 h per week with hobbies and recreation. Hence, it was not surprising that 56 % were dissatisfied with the amount of time available for family, and 81 % were dissatisfied with the amount of time available for hobbies and recreation. This problem was further compounded by the fact that from an average of 28 days per year of available vacation, only 20 days per year were effectively taken [23]. Similarly, in another national survey, half the surgeons felt that their work schedules did not allow enough time for their personal lives [18]. In yet another recent national survey, 64% (of nearly 8,000 sampled surgeons) felt that their work schedules did not leave enough time for personal and family life [19]. Similarly, a report from the American Pediatric Surgical Association Task Force on Family Issues noted that only 6% of practicing pediatric surgeons reported sufficient time for themselves, only 12% strongly disagreed with the statement "work has/had a detrimental effect on family life," and only 11% strongly agreed that they were able to "balance my professional and family responsibilities" [17]. These findings were further substantiated by the responses from their partners. Only 6% of the pediatric surgeons' partners strongly agreed with the statement "we rarely experience(d) conflict between…professional and family duties" [17].

Adverse Consequences of Work-Life Imbalance—Personal Level

A failed relationship, with or without divorce, may reflect inadequate time with, or attention towards, a spouse or significant other. In a survey of academic surgeons, two-thirds of the respondents reported that their demands at work "adversely affected their relationships with spouses" [24]. Interestingly, in comparing medical specialties, divorce rates tended to be among the highest for surgeons, with a reported 30% incidence over a 30-year time span [25]. Even after adjusting for other potentially confounding factors, being a surgeon conferred a relative risk of 1.7 for divorce, as compared with internists [25].

Excessive alcohol use may also be traced back to work-life imbalance in at least some surgeons. In a survey of members of the American College of Surgeons, 13.9% of all male and 25.6% of all female responding surgeons reported symptoms consistent with a diagnosis of alcohol abuse or alcohol dependence (could not fulfill their responsibilities because of drinking, were unable to stop drinking, were drinking in the morning, or were binge drinking) [8]. These surprisingly high incidences were corroborated in another longitudinal study of a large number of surgical graduates, 7.3% of whom had symptoms of alcohol dependence [6]. This alcohol dependence also contributed to practice attrition rates at these graduates' later career stages [6].

Other serious mental health issues such as depression and suicide can also be causally linked to work-life imbalance in at least some of the surgeons affected by these issues. In a large national survey, 30% of surgeons screened positive for depression [19]. Possibly as many as half of these surgeons would have qualified for a diagnosis of major depression if given a full psychiatric evaluation [19]. It is thus not surprising that a recent study among surgeons found a 6.3% rate of suicidal ideations during the previous 12 months [21]. Particularly for surgeons 45 years and older, this appeared to be a significant problem, as suicidal ideation was 1.5–3.0 times more common among surgeons than in the general population [21]. For the actual suicide incidence, no specific data about surgeons is available. In the overall physician population, though, male physicians' relative mortality ratio from suicide is already 1.5 to 3.8-fold higher than for their non-medical professional counterparts. In female physicians, the increased propensity for death from suicide is even greater with a 3.7 to 4.5-fold increased death rate from suicide [26–29].

Although not specifically studied for surgeons, chronic deterioration of physical health as manifested by hypertension, cardiovascular disease (including coronary artery disease), and sleep disorders, for instance, can also be indicators of the chronic inability to master the challenges between a demanding professional life and the need to maintain good somatic and mental health and at least a basic physical fitness [30, 31].

Adverse Consequences of Work-Life Imbalance—Professional Level

Suboptimal patient care and adverse patient outcomes may result from work-life imbalance. For instance, work-life imbalance has been causally associated with depression and burnout. The latter two conditions were shown to be independent predictors of the reporting of a major medical error by surgeons [20, 21].

Furthermore, when surgeons display emotional exhaustion, disengagement, hostility, or disruptive behavior towards patients, colleagues, and coworkers, there is a high likelihood that such behaviors are, at least in part, due to overwork and stress.

Many surgeons seek early retirement and may be motivated to do so because of difficulties with balancing work and life [22]. The reported median retirement age for surgeons is 57 years [32]. This is particularly impressive given that most surgeons have invested many years and considerable financial means into their education, residency and fellowship training, and into the establishment of their surgical practice. Consistent with those findings, a surprisingly large proportion (approximately 40%) of surgeons would not recommend their profession to their own children [19, 23, 33].

Adverse Consequences of Work-Life Imbalance—Personal and Professional Level: Burnout

Overwhelming stress and work-life imbalance can also lead to burnout, which encompasses and affects both personal and professional domains. Burnout is characterized by emotional exhaustion, depersonalization (treating patients and colleagues as objects rather than as human beings), and a decreased sense of personal accomplishment [34]. Burnout tends to be more common in human service occupations such as physicians, nurses, and social workers. Of all physicians, surgeons may be particularly prone to this syndrome due to the intensity of caring for their often very ill and complex patients, the high level of commitment and responsibilities of a surgical practice, the unpredictable and long hours (median hours worked per week according to a recent survey of US surgeons: 60 h), and the physical demands associated with the profession [23]. In the United States, according to several studies, up to 40% of all surgeons across all subspecialties are burned out [7, 8, 11–14, 19, 22]. Interestingly, a high prevalence of burnout among surgeons has also been reported from other countries. In a survey of the Young Fellows of the Royal Australasian College of Surgeons, 53% of all respondents reported high burnout levels (20% suffered work burnout, 27% suffered personal burnout, and 6% suffered patient burnout) [15, 16]. A similar study among colorectal and vascular surgeons from the United Kingdom reported high burnout scores for 31% of the respondents [10]. Burnout thus appears to not be associated with a particular culture or type of healthcare system.

According to the aforementioned studies, independent risk factors for burnout include age (younger > older), gender (women > men), unmarried status, age of children under 21 years, spouse in a health care profession, lack of spousal support, work-home conflict, poor work-life balance, lack of career satisfaction, area of specialization (highest in trauma surgery), poor professional relationships, perceived lack of supervisor support, lack of autonomy, number of nights on call per week, hours worked per week, nonacademic practice, hospital size <60 beds, and compensation based entirely on billing [7, 9–14, 19, 22, 35–37]. Not surprisingly, burnout was found to strongly correlate with the desire to retire early [22].

Prevention of and Recovery from Work-Life Imbalance

As with any medical problem, prevention is by far preferable to treatment. From a practical perspective, preventive and interventional/therapeutic measures overlap to a large extent and are often virtually indistinguishable. They will therefore be discussed jointly in this section.

"Know thyself" should always be the starting point. What is your heart telling you? What are your needs and your family's needs? What are your interests? What are your talents? What are your core values? What is your mission? What is your vision?

With regard to any personal or professional action plan, setting priorities and establishing realistic goals is paramount and derives directly from the aforementioned self-analysis. The following is intended to help in setting such priorities and goals, but it is ultimately up to each surgeon to ensure that these goals are realistic and appropriately tailored to individual life situations and professional circumstances.

Action Plan for Finding Balance and Decreasing Burnout—Personal Level

At a personal level, it is important to take the time to foster and nurture friendships and relationships. They can serve to "re-ground" and re-energize you, will enrich your non-work time and add meaning to your life. These relationships also provide a critical support system, especially during challenging phases of your life.

The relationship with the spouse or partner is the one that is most often neglected and taken for granted due to the limited free time in the surgical profession. Two-thirds of academic surgeons felt that the demands of work adversely affected their relationships with their spouses [24]. Women surgeons are even more likely than men to experience work-home conflicts [35]. The potential beneficial effects of limiting, or even reducing, work hours have been suggested by the results of a study of surgery residents after the introduction of the 80-h work week. Seventy-one percent of respondents noted that the quality of their relationships improved subsequent to the restriction of work hours [2, 38]. You must have specific "you and me" time with your spouse or partner. It is acceptable to use, at least occasionally, a babysitter or nanny to enjoy truly protected time together (e.g., "date nights"). When spending time with your spouse or partner, you must be rested and mentally present in order to be able to devote all attention to, and to make the most of, your joint time. This will strengthen, reinforce, and invigorate both the emotional and the physical aspects of your relationship.

Fixed family time must be built into the schedule. Important family events cannot be missed and must be prioritized. Multitasking (combined pursuit of work and home duties) at home must be—if not eliminated—at least severely restricted. When with the family, you must be 100 % present in mind and body and not pursue work-related tasks at the same time (except, for instance, when being on-call from home). If duties at home become too overwhelming, you should strongly consider hiring help with house chores and other routine duties in order to minimize avoidable stress and time not directly devoted to the family. Ideally, pastimes and hobbies should be chosen that allow for spending time with the family (e.g. hiking, skiing, music, chess playing, coaching child's sports team). Nonetheless, even chores, errands and other tasks that cannot be delegated to hired outside helpers can be viewed as opportunities to spend time together with the children. Vacation time should be reserved for true dedicated family vacations and not for attending medical meetings.

Imperfection around the house must be accepted, particularly at times when family demands are high, such as with younger children. The house does not always have to be spotless and you should heed the important tenet "Don't sweat the small stuff". Overall, it is paramount to be as invested in your spouse or partner and the children as you are invested in yourself and in your career.

The "me" aspect is often excluded from a personal action plan due to lack of time, attention, and priority, yet it is essential for an individual's well-being, too. Time for self-reflection and meditation is an important component of the maintenance of an adequate work-life balance. It is important to acknowledge that even with a very busy professional and family life, it is acceptable and necessary to have time for hobbies and personal interests, even if these involve only relatively short, but recurrent, time spans (e.g., reading a newspaper, learning a language). Many sports fulfill the needs of both physical and mental rejuvenation [9]. It is important to acknowledge that a fulfilled life outside of work enhances the insight into your patients' problems and helps you to better understand them [39].

Personal health must be optimized. This involves maintenance of an active exercise schedule, intake of good nutrition, and provision of sufficient sleep. Optimization of personal health should also include seeking adequate preventive medical care and establishing a relationship with a primary care physician. According to a recent survey of members of the American College of Surgeons, only about half of the responding surgeons did pursue a regular physical exercise schedule and only 46 % had seen a primary care provider over the preceding 12 months—indicating ample room for improvement of practices in these two areas of personal wellness [9]. Prompt attention should be sought for any physical or mental health issues. Unfortunately, surgeons (and other physicians) tend to be reluctant to seek psychiatric or psychological help when needed. Among surgeons with suicidal ideations, for instance, only 26 % had sought professional help over the preceding 12 months, and 60 % reported that they were reluctant to seek such help because of the concern that it might adversely affect their license to practice medicine [21].

For the achievement and maintenance of an adequate mental balance, time must also be made for the pursuit of specific spiritual, religious, or meditation practices in accordance with personal beliefs.

In trying to incorporate and maintain the above recommendations into your schedule, it is of utmost importance to acknowledge that their implementation will require active (re)scheduling, active protection of time, and ongoing monitoring. Otherwise, work-related elements frequently creep back into the daily schedule.

Action Plan for Finding Balance and Decreasing Burnout—Professional Level

All actions taken at the personal and family level in order to achieve work-life balance must be mirrored by corresponding actions at the professional level. The characterization of a physician from a previous generation as "He was always overworked and proud of it" has become anachronistic and appears completely out of place in today's surgical work environment [40]. There is a fine line separating dedication from over-work. Again, thorough self-analysis at the outset is important to allow you to match your competencies, interests and available time to the demands of your particular position. You must be ready to adjust your expectations.

When looking at potential surgical positions and practices, you should choose a position, practice, or group that shares your values and respects your and others' boundaries, and is able to appreciate your talents and contributions. During the interview process, these needs must be kept in mind. Are there surgical hospitalists? Who covers call? What are call and work-hour requirements? How flexible is the workplace? Is childcare available at the workplace (as already offered by some institutions)? What is the flexibility regarding potential part-time positions should children be added to the family? What is the maternity and paternity leave policy?

Identifying and focusing on areas at work to which you can contribute most, and from which you can derive the most meaning and gratification (e.g., research vs. clinical care vs. medical education vs. administrative tasks), is an important strategy. Also positive-psychology self-interventions have been shown to enhance subjective and psychological well-being, to help reduce depressive symptoms, and to be associated with multiple other beneficial emotional and interpersonal benefits. Such self-interventions include placing greater emphasis on finding meaning in work, focusing on what is important in life, maintaining a positive outlook, embracing a philosophy that stresses work-life balance, practicing gratitude by counting one's blessings (as opposed to burdens) and by keeping a (daily or weekly) gratitude journal (positive writing), positive future thinking and projecting a positive self in the future, as well as use of online intervention options [41, 42].

Minimizing all non-essential activities is critical. The latter may involve prioritizing your commitments to local, regional, and national committees and organizations. It is difficult, if not impossible, to actively participate in multiple committees and societies at the same time and to significantly contribute to each one. Not infrequently, increasing your focus will require a certain amount of callousness in order to be able to let go of certain tasks and duties. In the current era, it is particularly important to acknowledge that you cannot be a master in all areas. The "quadruple threat" status may be *de facto* unattainable by many of the currently practicing surgeons given the expectations, complexity and rigors of the surgical field. Overall, it is important to remind yourself periodically that at work *everybody* is replaceable. Nonetheless, cherish and appreciate your position.

Besides focusing and restricting the scope of the work, consideration should be given to obtaining additional training or undergoing re-training and/or changing the work focus. Such measures may help decrease stress if, as a result, you are able to work in a targeted and focused area in which you can excel and/or that may allow for more flexibility, or even a decrease of the work hours.

When at work, you must be highly organized and efficient. In that regard, we refer to the chapter elsewhere in this book that is specifically dedicated to optimizing time management. Regardless of the practices adopted to optimize time management, it is important to learn to delegate and to trust those to whom work is delegated. This involves employing only judiciously selected people, and then continuously developing them. Look for colleagues who are able to achieve balance themselves and try to learn from them.

For implementation of any of the above measures, a culture of open communication with the departmental chair or divisional chief is important. This will allow the surgical leadership to better understand stressful aspects and challenges of routine clinical and research business, and may be instrumental in helping to devise and implement remedial measures as necessary. Moreover, an open communication culture among colleagues allows for discussion and debriefing after adverse clinical outcomes (e.g., patient death), which have been shown to be risk factors for distress and psychological imbalance [21].

The recommendations discussed in this section can be difficult to execute as many of them require a change of individual mindset and culture, particularly when it comes to patient care-related changes.

Conclusion

When trying to balance personal and work life, it is important to acknowledge that there is no generally applicable blueprint. Work-life balance is different for different individuals and, like an ever-swinging pendulum, may be different for the same person at different times in his or her life. Given the demands and constraints of the current work environment, surgeons must be able to draw from a broad repertoire of wellness promotion practices (many of which have been outlined above) in order to achieve high well-being and work-life balance. Striving for that balance requires ongoing follow-up, monitoring and adjustment as needed. Regardless of the pathway you choose, it would be a fallacy, however, to get caught up in the belief that your personal life can be placed on hold indefinitely or until retirement. The latter is a mistake that appears to be all too often committed by surgeons, particularly by those who over-invest themselves in their professional lives.

Besides the measures that individual surgeons can take to prevent or correct work-life imbalance and related problems, such as burnout, the surgical profession as a whole (surgeons, academic and nonacademic departments and institutions, and professional societies) must advocate for, and work towards, effecting change at the surgical workplace. Such necessary change includes creation of more part-time and other flexible surgical work opportunities, broader implementation of shift work for surgeons (as has already occurred in some hospitals and in some subspecialties [e.g., trauma surgery]), the creation of surgical hospitalist positions, and increasing the availability of childcare at the workplace. Although these proposals may sound far-fetched to some, other countries have already moved on even further. For instance, in the Netherlands, the concept of part-time work has now also permeated to the level of surgical training [43]. As stated by a Dutch medical leader ("…if we insisted on full-time surgeons, we would have a personnel problem"), such considerations are not a luxury, but may turn into a necessity in the not too distant future [43].

Ultimately, it is only the combination of mindful effort and goal setting at the personal and professional level, coupled with focused institutional, national and societal surgical advocacy that will change how surgeons can cope with challenges of maintaining physical and emotional health in the face of the ever increasing complexities and demands of their profession. A change in surgical culture, including acceptance of the fact that it is appropriate to talk about work-life imbalance issues and burnout, will result in a better and more sustainable lifestyle for surgeons. Such change benefits not only individual surgeons, but also surgical departments and patients, since work-life imbalance and burnout are risk factors for underperformance at work and medical errors.

Appropriate attention to these matters will help you to better enjoy and appreciate the innumerable rewards and gratifications that can be derived from the surgical profession. Implementation of at least some of the recommendations discussed in this chapter will also make you a better spouse, parent, friend, surgeon, colleague, mentor, educator, and researcher. If you are able to balance your life, the legacy you will leave behind will be far greater in its impact and influence on your family, patients, and the surgical community.

References

1. Blaisdell FW. Development of the city-county (public) hospital. Arch Surg. 1994;129(7):760–4.
2. Irani JL, Mello MM, Ashley SW, Whant EE, Zinner MJ, Breen E. Surgical residents' perceptions of the effects of the ACGME duty hour requirements 1 year after implementation. Surgery. 2005;138(2):246–53.
3. Fischer JE. Continuity of care: a casualty of the 80-hour work week. Acad Med. 2004;79(5):381–3.
4. Vanderveen K, Bold RJ. Effect of generational composition on the surgical workforce. Arch Surg. 2008;143(3):224–6.
5. Troppmann KM, Palis BE, Goodnight Jr JE, Ho HS, Troppmann C. Women surgeons in the new millennium. Arch Surg. 2009;144(7):635–42.
6. Harms BA, Heise CP, Gould JC, Starling JR. A 25-year single institution analysis of health, practice, and fate of general surgeons. Ann Surg. 2005;242(4):520–9.
7. Johnson JT, Wagner RL, Rueger RM, Goepfert H. Professional burnout among head and neck surgeons: results of a survey. Head Neck. 1993;15(6):557–60.
8. Oreskovich MR, Kaups KL, Balch CM, Hanks JB, Satele D, Sloan J, Meredith C, Buhl A, Dyrbye LN, Shanafelt TD. Prevalence of alcohol use disorders among American surgeons. Arch Surg. 2012;147(2):168–74.
9. Shanafelt TD, Oreskovich MR, Dyrbye LN, Satele DV, Hanks JB, Sloan JA, Balch CM. Avoiding burnout: the personal health habits and wellness practices of US surgeons. Ann Surg. 2012;255(4):625–33.
10. Sharma A, Sharp DM, Walker LG, Monson JR. Stress and burnout in colorectal and vascular surgical consultants working in the UK National Health Service. Psychooncology. 2008;17(6):570–6.
11. Balch CM, Shanafelt TD, Sloan JA, Satele DV, Freischlag JA. Distress and career satisfaction among 14 surgical specialties, comparing academic and private practice settings. Ann Surg. 2011;254(4):558–68.
12. Jesse MT, Abouljoud M, Eshelman A. Determinants of burnout among transplant surgeons: a national survey in the United States. Am J Transplant. 2015;15(3):772–8.
13. Balch CM, Freischlag JA, Shanafelt TD. Stress and burnout among surgeons: Understanding and managing the syndrome and avoiding the adverse consequences. Arch Surg. 2009;144(4):371–6.
14. Balch CM, Shanafelt T. Combating stress and burnout in surgical practice: a review. Adv Surg. 2010;44:29–47.
15. Benson S, Truskett PG, Findlay B. The relationship between burnout and emotional intelligence in Australian surgeons and surgical trainees. ANZ J Surg. 2007;77 suppl 1:A79.
16. Benson S, Sammour T, Neuhaus SJ, Findlay B, Hill AG. Burnout in Australasian younger fellows. ANZ J Surg. 2009;79(9):590–7.
17. Katz A, Mallory B, Gilbert JC, Bethel C, Hayes-Jordan AA, Saito JM, et al. State of the practice for pediatric surgery—career satisfaction and concerns. A report from the American Pediatric Surgical Association Task Force on Family Issues. J Pediatr Surg. 2010;45(10):1975–82.
18. Schroen AT, Brownstein MR, Sheldon GF. Comparison of private versus academic practice for general surgeons: a guide for medical students and residents. J Am Coll Surg. 2003;197(6):1000–11.

19. Shanafelt TD, Balch CM, Bechamps GJ, Russell T, Dyrbye L, Satele D, et al. Burnout and career satisfaction among American surgeons. Ann Surg. 2009;250(3):463–71.
20. Shanafelt TD, Balch CM, Bechamps G, Russell T, Dyrbye L, Satele D, et al. Burnout and medical errors among American surgeons. Ann Surg. 2010;251(6):995–1000.
21. Shanafelt TD, Balch CM, Dyrbye L, Bechamps G, Russell T, Satele D, et al. Special report: suicidal ideation among American surgeons. Arch Surg. 2011;146(1):54–62.
22. Campbell Jr DA, Sonnad SS, Eckhauser FE, Campbell KK, Greenfield LJ. Burnout among American surgeons. Surgery. 2001;130940:696–705.
23. Troppmann KM, Palis BE, Goodnight JE, Ho HS, Troppmann C. Career and lifestyle satisfaction among surgeons: what really matters? The National Lifestyles in Surgery Today Survey. J Am Coll Surg. 2009;209(2):160–9.
24. Colletti LM, Mulholland MW, Sonnad SS. Perceived obstacles to career success for women in academic surgery. Arch Surg. 2000;135(8):972–7.
25. Rollman BL, Mead LA, Wang N-Y, Klag MJ. Medical specialty and the incidence of divorce. N Engl J Med. 1997;336(11):800–3.
26. Center C, Davis M, Detre T, Ford DE, Hansbrough W, Hendin H, et al. Confronting depression and suicide in physicians: a consensus statement. JAMA. 2003;289(23):3161–6.
27. Frank E, Biola H, Burnett CA. Mortality rates and causes among U.S. physicians. Am J Prev Med. 2000;19(3):155–9.
28. Frank E, Dingle AD. Self-reported depression and suicide attempts among U.S. women physicians. Am J Psychiatry. 1999;156(12):1887–94.
29. Lindeman S, Laara E, Hakko H, Lonnqvist J. A systematic review on gender-specific suicide mortality in medical doctors. Br J Psychiatry. 1996;168(3):274–9.
30. Ford DE, Mead LA, Chang PP, Cooper-Patrick L, Wang NY, Klag MJ. Depression is a risk factor for coronary artery disease in men: the precursors study. Arch Intern Med. 1998;158(13):1422–6.
31. Lundberg U. Stress hormones in health and illness: the roles of work and gender. Psychoneuroendocrinology. 2005;30(10):1017–21.
32. Association of American Medical Colleges. AAMC data book: statistical information related to medical schools and teaching hospitals. Washington: AAMC; 2001.
33. Kibbe MR, Troppmann C, Barnett Jr CC, Nwomeh BC, Olutoye OO, Doria C, et al. Effect of educational debt on career and quality of life among academic surgeons. Ann Surg. 2009;249(2):342–8.
34. Maslach C, Jackson SE, Leiter MP. MBI: the maslach burnout inventory: manual. Palo Alto: Consulting Psychologists Press; 1996.
35. Dyrbye LN, Shanafelt TD, Balch CM, Satele D, Sloan J, Freischlag J. Relationship between work-home conflicts and burnout among American surgeons: a comparison by sex. Arch Surg. 2011;146(2):211–7.
36. Ng TW, Sorensen KL. Toward a further understanding of the relationships between perceptions of support and work attitudes: a meta-analysis. Group Organization Management 2008; 33(3):243–68.
37. Oskrochi Y, Maruthappu M, Henriksson M, Davies AH, Shalhoub J. Beyond the body: a systematic review of the nonphysical effects of a surgical career. Surgery. 2016;159(2):650–64.
38. Powell AC, Nelson JS, Massarweh NN, Brewster LP, Santry HP. The modern surgical lifestyle. Bull Am Coll Surg. 2009;96(6):33–7.
39. Charon R. Narrative medicine: honoring stories of illness. Oxford: Oxford University Press; 2007.
40. Berger J. A fortunate man: the story of a country doctor. New York: Random House; 1997.
41. Emmons RA, McCullough ME. Counting blessings versus burdens: an experimental investigation of gratitude and subjective well-being in daily life. J Pers Soc Psychol. 2003;84(2):377–89.
42. Bolier L, Haverman M, Westerhof GJ, Riper H, Smit P, Bohlmeijer E. Positive psychology interventions: a meta-analysis of randomized controlled studies. BMC Public Health. 2013;13:119.
43. Bennhold K. Flexible workweek alters the rhythm of Dutch life: Going part time appeals to both sexes. The New York Times; Dec 30, 2010, p. A10.

Chapter 15
Time Management

Carla M. Pugh and Jay N. Nathwani

Introduction

Becoming a successful faculty member in an academic medical center is not a trivial undertaking. Success requires strong effort in three major areas including patient care, teaching, and research. A commonality amongst the great achievers in academia, and other professions, is excellent time management skills. While no one is born knowing how to prepare and deliver effective scientific presentations; write a successful research grant; build a world-class research program; manage research assistants; and balance the endless and often conflicting time demands imposed by clinical practice, teaching, research, and administrative service – a time management plan will greatly facilitate achievement in these areas.

Time management has been defined as the use of a set of principles, practices, skills, and tools to accomplish specific tasks and goals. It is important to note that time management is a broad subject that covers many different areas from day-to-day actions to long-term goals. A good time management system integrates several skills including planning, prioritizing, goal setting, scheduling, and maximizing efficiency. The goal is to have a consistent set of tools designed to work well with each other. The principles and practices involved in time management are broad and

C.M. Pugh (✉) • J.N. Nathwani
Department of Surgery, University of Wisconsin-Madison,
School of Medicine and Public Health,
Madison, WI, USA

heavily dependent on your personal goals, specialty, and academic setting. This chapter provides an overview of the most successful time management strategies available. Examples on how to use these strategies for common academic tasks, projects, and goals are provided.

Time Management Strategies

Figure 15.1 provides a list of the most important time management strategies and associated topics. Time management has become an extremely popular subject due to the ever-increasing desire for efficiency and work-life balance. Whether you search the Internet or visit the self-help section of the local book store you will inevitably find numerous resources – some helpful, some not. The best chance of choosing the one that is right for you is to conduct a personal inventory of your time management skills (Fig. 15.2). Once you understand where you are in the process of achieving excellent time management skills, you will be better equipped to reach the next level.

Which scenario best describes you?

Fig. 15.1 Key time management strategies

Planning and prioritizing	Scheduling Protected time
To do lists Saying "NO" Action plans Activity logs	Eliminating distractions Writing/reading days Buffer time Email
Goal setting	**Maximizing efficiency**
Completing large tasks 1-, 5- and 10-year goals The big picture	Getting organized Multitasking Positive thinking

Fig. 15.2 Time management assessment

Scenario 1	Scenario 2
Are you completely overwhelmed because you have a failing strategy?	*Do you already have a strategy in place and are looking to improve it?*
This chapter will help you to understand the basics of time management and get started with implementing a plan	This chapter will help you better understand the terminology needed to perform focused searches for specific strategies that will lead to improvement

Fig. 15.3 Useful tips for planning and prioritizing

> **USEFUL TIPS FOR PLANNING AND PRIORITIZING**
>
> Make big plans for daily achievement. You are likely to accomplish more. Book everything as an appointment.
>
> Apply the 80/20 rule - The 80/20 rule states that 20% of your tasks account for 80% of the value in your to-do list. Some tasks have a much greater return on your investment of time and energy than others. Use prioritization to identify and focus your time on these high-payoff tasks.
>
> Take the time to plan your week and forecast what your week will look like. Put aside thirty minutes Sunday night or Monday morning to plan your routine or develop a list of what needs to be accomplished during the week.
>
> "The best planning strategy is to do ugliest thing first." Dr. Randy Pausch

TO-DO LISTS	Sample List 1 Simple	Sample List 2 Prioritized	Sample List 3 Partitioned
Write it down. A common mistake is to try to use your memory to keep track of too many details. This can lead to information overload. Writing things down is a great way to take control of your projects and tasks to keep yourself organized.	Email Mary ~~Call Tom~~ ~~Finalize Travel~~ Book chapter images Start lit review New cell phone charger	~~1- Finalize Travel~~ ~~1- Call Tom~~ 1- New cell phone charger 2- Email Mary 2- Book chapter images 3- Start lit review	**Major** ~~1- Finalize Travel (30 min)~~ 2- Book chapter images (2 hrs) 3- Start lit review (1 hr) **Minor** ~~1- Call Tom~~ 1- New cell phone charger 2- Email Mary
Prioritize. Prioritizing your to-do list helps you focus and spend more of your time on the things that really matter. Rate your tasks into categories using a prioritization system that is meaning ful to you.	**Comment:** Better than nothing, but should be prioritized	**Comment:** Numbers, days, or times can help add priority	**Comment:** Can facilitate multi-tasking (ie. Call Tom while searching for images)

Fig. 15.4 Sample to-do lists

Planning and Prioritizing

Planning and prioritizing go hand-in-hand and are perhaps the most important time management strategies (Fig. 15.3). Simply scheduling how your day would go and prioritizing the day using a to-do list will help make sure that you can get your tasks completed. It is advisable to list both the things you want to accomplish and the allotted time for completion (Fig. 15.4). This ensures a complete list and facilitates staying on time.

Delegating and Saying "No"

Keep in mind that you cannot (and should not) do everything. If you think you have too many tasks on hand, delegate. Goal setting and mentors can greatly facilitate your ability to delegate and to say "no"; Fig. 15.5 depicts the Urgency-Importance

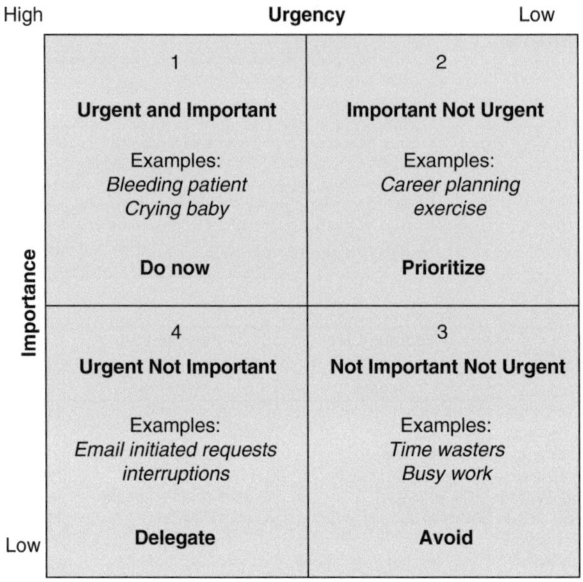

	High	Urgency	Low
Importance High	**1** **Urgent and Important** Examples: *Bleeding patient* *Crying baby* **Do now**	**2** **Important Not Urgent** Examples: *Career planning exercise* **Prioritize**	
Importance Low	**4** **Urgent Not Important** Examples: *Email initiated requests interruptions* **Delegate**	**3** **Not Important Not Urgent** Examples: *Time wasters* *Busy work* **Avoid**	

Fig. 15.5 The urgency-importance matrix (Adapted from Birshan [1])

Matrix. Delegation should not be viewed as off-loading work. While you may be competent to follow through on a requested project, whether or not it is a good use of your time may be the prevailing question. Sharing opportunities with the right mentee may help develop a young academic career. The key to successful delegation is choosing a recipient who is capable to complete the task. In the process of delegation, one should be careful to still plan and oversee the work [6]. Supervision of the work allows you to ensure a high quality end product and allows for the opportunity to develop your mentee's abilities by providing guidance and support.

Excepting a few clinical specialties, high-urgency, high-importance events are rare. Everything else can be planned. Keeping a list of your daily, monthly, and annual priorities handy can help you decide what to accept, delegate, or reject. Although there will invariably be situations where you find it difficult to say no, there are key strategies to handling this as well (Fig. 15.6). It is imperative that you learn to say, "no". Quality of work is often more important than quantity.

Action Plans

While to-do lists are great for managing daily and weekly tasks, action plans capture the big picture. Action plans help you keep track of your progress toward achieving short-, medium-, and long-term goals. The necessary steps in creating an action plan include: (1) clarifying your goals; (2) writing a list of actions; (3) analyzing and prioritizing the list; and (4) documenting the planned execution details

The Difficult "NO"

Common Scenarios	General Approach
These will invariably happen when: 1) you are completing your first R-01, 2) have a busy travel schedule, or 3) you are already overwhelmed	*Any of these approaches may be visible options for addressing the common scenarios presented.*
You are invited to your first visiting professorship	**Before you respond:**
Prestigious organization X asks you to be on a committee	Check your ego
	Consult your list of priorities & strategic goals
	Consult your mentor
Your Division Chief offers your name as someone who is perfect and available for a task that has national recognition	Have a clear plan (with options)
	In your response:
	Be profusely thankful
The Dean's office nominates you for a task or committee	Openly recognize the importance of the task
	Openly recognize the importance of the invitation
Several of your collaborators team up to apply for a major grant of interest in your area	<u>Negotiate</u>: Is it possible to do it next year?
	Can you delegate an insider?
You are invited to be a keynote speaker	<u>Saying "No"</u>:
	Be open & honest (the invitor will appreciate it)
	"I have an R-01 due that day"
	"I am unable to take on additional tasks"

Fig. 15.6 Useful tips for saying "no"

(what, who, where, when, and how). The most common tool used in making an action plan explicit is a white board. Get one. Several project management software tools have this capability as well.

Activity Logs

Activity logs are time management learning tools. If you are really struggling with time management, this is an extremely useful exercise. The best way to start the log is to plan the night before how you will document your activities. To get the best detail, plan to write down everything you do on a 30-min time scale. This can be done on a sheet of paper or by using your smart device. Try to update it every 1–2 h. Most people are surprised how they spend their time. This activity can help motivate you to prioritize, schedule protected blocks of time, and manage relationships. Tables 15.1 and 15.2 [2] list common time wasters and useful time savers.

Scheduling Protected Time

Emails, telephone calls, meetings, and administrative tasks can fill your schedule and make you inefficient if you allow it. Grouping like tasks on the same day will increase your chances of being able to have protected time for reading and writing (Fig. 15.7). For example, if you have two clinical days per week combined with three research

Table 15.1 Common time wasters

Worrying about it and putting it off, which leads to indecision
Creating inefficiency by implementing first instead of analyzing first
Unanticipated interruptions that do not pay off
Procrastinating
Making unrealistic time estimates
Unnecessary errors (not enough time to do it right, but enough time to do it over)
Crisis management
Poor organization
Ineffective meetings
Micromanaging by failing to let others perform and grow
Doing urgent rather than important tasks
Poor planning and lack of contingency plans
Failing to delegate
Lacking priorities, standards, policies, and procedures

From Clark [2]; with permission

Table 15.2 Useful time savers

Managing the decision-making process, not the decisions
Concentrating on doing only one task at a time
Establishing daily, short-term, mid-term, and long-term priorities
Handling correspondence expeditiously with quick, short letters and memos
Throwing unneeded things away
Establishing personal deadlines and ones for the organization
Not wasting other people's time
Ensuring all meetings have a purpose, time limit, and include only essential people
Getting rid of busywork
Maintaining accurate calendars; abide by them
Knowing when to stop a task, policy, or procedure
Delegating everything possible and empowering subordinates
Keeping things simple
Ensuring time is set aside to accomplish high-priority tasks
Setting aside time for reflection
Using checklists and to-do lists
Adjusting priorities as a result of new tasks

From Clark [2]; with permission

days, it works better if you can have your clinical days back to back (preferably Monday-Tuesday or Thursday-Friday). This will enable better control of your schedule and increase the likelihood that you can schedule protected time (i.e. Tuesdays for scientific writing). The more diligent and consistent you are about your protected time, the easier it will be to institute an action plan and meet your goals.

> **USEFUL TIPS WHEN PROTECTING TIME**
>
> *"Find your creative time and defend it ruthlessly."* Dr. Randy Pausch
>
> *"Plan an hour per day for 'Me Time'. Give twenty-three hours to the world but keep one hour for yourself."* Dr. Donald Wetmore
>
> *When negotiating your schedule, group like activities (i.e. 2 clinical days followed by 3 research days). This will help you to compartmentalize your tasks.*
>
> *Be purposeful in generating a culture of protected research time. A closed door on Tuesdays will send the message that this is a "do not disturb" day*

Fig. 15.7 Useful tips when protecting time

Eliminating Distractions

It is important for you to identify the things that distract you. This will enable you to work on ways to minimize or completely eliminate distractions. You may be surprised how much work you can finish in an hour of uninterrupted time. In addition, you should resist the urge to distract yourself with other things. Try hard to finish one task before jumping to another. In other words, chain yourself to the task chair. If you find yourself struggling with this, it may be that you have not broken the task into achievable units. The more you are able to fully concentrate and commit to the work you are doing in a scheduled time period, the faster you will be able to complete the task. Finding a hide-out may greatly facilitate this.

Buffer Time

In addition to underestimating the time it will take you to complete a task, there are several things that will invariably pop up or intrude on your scheduled time. Planning for the unexpected is a helpful way to keep yourself on time and on target toward meeting your goals. When working on large tasks such as a research project or grant, plan for failed experiments, late equipment, computer viruses, or writer's block. When traveling during the winter months, it is always helpful to build in a day or two of buffer time between your planned return and important face-to-face meetings. Rescheduling important meetings wastes everyone's time. Not only do you have to inform everyone that you will miss the meeting, you then have to repeat the process of reviewing meeting materials and goals and finding available dates, conference rooms, etc. Other unexpected events commonly include family emergencies, home and car emergencies, and unplanned personal health issues. Having the buffer time keeps you less stressed and on time.

Email

Whether you are working online or using your smart device, it is tempting to check email every minute or every hour. This is a form of distraction that can significantly hinder task completion. Tables 15.3 and 15.4 [3, 4] provide several tips for those who are addicted to email and time-saving advice for those wishing to manage email more effectively.

Goal Setting

We desire efficient and effective time management because we want to reach our goals (Fig. 15.8). The process of goal setting relates to directing your conscious and subconscious decisions toward success and building motivation to achieve your goals. The SMART concept states that your goals should be: (1) **S**pecific, (2) **M**easureable, (3) **A**ttainable, (4) **R**ewarding, and (5) **T**imely (Table 15.5) [5].

Completing Large Tasks

Many times we find ourselves in situations where we have to get something done, but we either do not enjoy the task, do not have the resources (e.g., time, knowledge, energy), or we simply just do not want to do it; but it has to get done. Whatever the

Table 15.3 Tips for those addicted to email

Some addiction signs
You check your email more than once an hour
You look at every message that comes in, as it comes in
You feel the need to respond to messages instantly or within minutes of when they arrive
You interrupt real, in-person activities on a regular basis to deal with email
Email has, in some way, interfered with your regular life (e.g., stress, sleep loss, relationship troubles, etc.)
Useful advice
There's no such thing as an email emergency. If something is incredibly urgent, the sender will call, text, or otherwise reach you
Give yourself a curfew. Decide on a specific cut-off time for sending and reading messages, and stick to it
Schedule email times. Set specific times during which you'll deal with email, and don't do it outside of those windows
Set aside a "no email" day. If you can't cope with taking a full day off, try only checking your email for 5 min on Saturday morning – then leaving the rest of the day email free
Turn your smart device off when you get home, or at least disable the instant email checking function. Your messages will wait, but your life will not

Adapted from Raphael [3]

Table 15.4 Time-saving email management strategies

1. Think before you write. Before you begin composing an email, consider what you're trying to accomplish and whether email is effective for your task. For example, if you're trying to solve someone's problem, call them instead
2. Keep it simple. Email works best for simple requests and messages that can be expressed within a few lines. If your message is going to necessitate more than two email chains, a phone call can save lots of time
3. Keep it short. People like email because it's fast and easy. However, the longer and more complicated your message, the longer it takes you to compose or respond
4. Make your subject line work. To help your recipient prioritize and understand your needs, your subject line should be very clear. Deadlines and dates in the subject line are very useful
5. Structure your email. There should be an opening, a body, and end. Sentences should be 15 words or less. Three or more points should be bulleted
6. Take ownership of your message. Ask the recipient. "Is there anything I can do to help? Did I give you enough information?"
7. Avoid words and phrases that make people defensive. Provoking words such as, "Why did you …," "You must…," "I'm sure you'll agree…," and "I don't understand your …," often indicate a breakdown in communication that cannot be remedied efficiently by email
8. Selectively use blind copy and reply all. The only reason to use blind copy is to keep your recipients' email address private. Don't use blind copy to surreptitiously share confidential or incriminating information with someone else. Replying to everyone can unnecessarily create inefficiency and email clutter for other people

Adapted from Levinson [4]

USEFUL TIPS FOR GOAL SETTING

Completing large tasks - Let the action be the reward. Once you have outlined a path, allow the doing or the process to be the reward and where the pleasure resides, not just the end result.

Break the mold - The key force that either drives you towards your goals or holds you back is your subconscious mind. Goal setting is necessary for your subconscious mind to accept your goals and start working for you. Otherwise it will work hard to keep you in the comfort zone of present conditions and old habits.

Fig. 15.8 Useful tips for goal setting

reason for the overwhelming feelings that persist during these times, the best approach is to divide the task into manageable parts. There are three useful steps in dividing large tasks:

1. **Identify the activities associated with the final completion of the task.** Brainstorm what needs to be done to complete the task. Sit down and write out the steps necessary to complete the task. Identification of key subtasks will help build a clear picture of the steps you need to take.
2. **Allocate time for subtasks.** Take your list of actions or subtasks and begin allocating time and dates to complete them. Try not to overburden yourself or you will resort to where you started and risk loss of motivation.

Table 15.5 SMART goals

Specific	Establishing a specific goal enables you to clarify what you want to achieve, and to set standards for that achievement. In making your goals specific, it is important that you *write them down*. This is crucial in all goal setting guidelines
Measurable	For a goal to be measurable you need a way to evaluate progress and document specific criteria that will tell you when you can stop and the goal is achieved. Being able to *document progress* is very important in staying motivated and is the key to enjoying the process of achieving the goal
Attainable	An attainable goal is a goal for which you *see a realistic path to achievement*, and know there are reasonable odds that you will get there. It is well known that the best goals provide a personal challenge. Succeeding at a challenging goal will give you more motivation and sense of achievement
Rewarding	You should have clear reasons why you want to reach a certain goal. It is important that the goal is really yours and that you can *clearly identify why achieving it will be rewarding for you*. This will help you stay motivated through difficult moments and not quit
Timely	Your goal should *have a specific time limit*. Time is the price you pay for the reward of achieving a goal. Setting the deadline will protect you from paying a higher price than the goal is worth. This can help protect you from procrastination and perfectionism

Adapted from Time-Management-Guide.com [5]

3. **Execution of subtasks.** At this point you should have a fairly clear picture of what needs to be done and how long it is going to take. Once you get started, keep in mind that each subtask you complete should give you a sense of accomplishment. This helps to keep you motivated and on target toward achieving the larger goal.

Maximizing Efficiency

The key to maximizing efficiency is being organized, multitasking when possible, and keeping a clear, positive drive toward meeting your goals (Fig. 15.9).

Get Organized

You can waste a lot of time during your day due to disorganization. Looking for documents, important emails, or previously used journal articles can easily steal hours of your time. Many people struggle with disorganization. While some think they can succeed amidst the chaos, disorganization has a high price. Lack of organization can hold you back from achieving your goals, block creativity, add stress to your life, and prevent you from being productive and effective.

> **USEFUL TIPS FOR MAXIMIZING EFFICIENCY**
>
> We can all afford to step back and ask if we are managing cur time properly and efficiently.
>
> Take a team apporach – ask for help, pay for help, invest time in training others to help.
>
> Personal health - "Some of it is part of who we are… we are naturally driven… but sometimes you have to get off the adrenaline train and reconnoiter…" Anonymous Professor
>
> Go to bed! – If you are tired, you are less likely to be productive.

Fig. 15.9 Useful tips for maximizing efficiency

Improving Your Daily Efficiency

Even with a full day of operating room cases and meetings, one can still improve efficiency. Many surgeons look at a long day of cases and meetings and concede that there is no time for additional work. The key is recognizing downtime and identifying which work tasks are eligible for the time allowed. Before and after each operating room case, one often finds that there is some downtime. Before the case the surgeon waits for the patient, support staff, and induction of anesthesia in the operating room. After the case, the surgeon waits for room turnover and a reoccurrence of the above process. This valuable downtime is often unrecognized as an opportunity to complete work. The key to completing work within these pockets of time is pinpointing the work that requires long periods of concentration and the work that can be easily picked up from the time last left off. There may be tasks that you may find suitable to work on in such an environment including editing papers, writing letters of support, or composing medical student reviews. Plan what work you will take with you. Even consider organizing a separate, pre-packed bag you could take with you when anticipating such downtime.

Multitasking

There are two camps when it comes to advice on multitasking – the true believers and the naysayers. Examples from the believer camp include deleting mass and spam emails that do not apply to you while riding an exercise bike in the gym or having multiple journal articles at various stages of completion. The naysayers believe multitasking makes you lose your focus and risks not getting any work done. Having multiple unfinished tasks creates stress for some people, but prevents boredom for others.

Think Positive

Worrying about your goals and tasks steals energy and wastes time. Whether you are questioning your ability to meet your goals or worrying about the acceptance of a paper or abstract, negative thoughts steal time away from other tasks. None of the time management strategies will work if you are distracted by negative thoughts. In fact there is now a fair amount of online training and support for *attention management* and *mindfulness*. These strategies can help you to maximize your energy and minimized wasted time. Another useful strategy is to talk to someone. Spouses, colleagues, and friends can help you address your concerns efficiently and help you get back on track. Dr. Donald Wetmore, a time management expert states:

> When you are in a negative mood you tend to repel the positive people who do not want to be strained and drained and brought down by your negativity. And, when you are in a negative mood, you have a natural system set up to attract the other negative people to you who want to share their stories of their misery so the two of you can compare experiences to decide who has the worse life. Positive people help to bring us up. Negative people help to bring us down.

Finding Your Equilibrium

With the demands that can be associated with a career in academics, it can be easy to lose sight of other important responsibilities. Without appropriate balance, hobbies, family, and friendships could be forgotten and neglected. Identifying and maintaining the aspects that are important to you could come with ease with the appropriate strategy. Establish daily habits to help maintain your work life balance. Block a small period of time daily to talk with family over dinner or pursue a hobby. Recognizing which events may be important to you is the first step to making sure that you can be a part of it. If you know of an important family event, for example, place it in your academic calendar as soon the date is announced. By marking important events on your academic calendar, you can ensure that a personal event will not be missed by a competing academic event.

Summary

A good time management system integrates several skills including planning, prioritizing, goal setting, scheduling, and maximizing efficiency. Maximizing efficiency requires mindfulness and attention management. The goal is to have a consistent set of tools that work well together. If you are new to time management, a useful approach is to identify your biggest problems first and start working on them. Time management cannot be mastered in just one sitting. In addition, as your goals evolve you will need new strategies. With continued refinement, you will master these strategies and get things done flawlessly and on time.

References

1. Birshan E. I am not perfect. Eitan Birshan dotcom. www.eitanbirshan.com/blog/page/6/. Accessed 1 Apr 2016.
2. Clark D. Time management for leaders. http://www.nwlink.com/~donclark/leader/leadtime.html. Accessed 1 Apr 2016.
3. Raphael JR. E-mail addiction: five signs it's time for an intervention. CIO. Published 12 Sept 2008. www.cio.com/article/449070/E_Mail_Addiction_Five_Signs_It_s_Time_for_an_Intervention. Accessed 1 Apr 2016.
4. Levinson M. E-mail etiquette: eight tips to avoid communication blunders. CIO. Published 19 May 2010. www.cio.com/article/594267/E_mail_Etiquette_8_Tips_to_Avoid_Communication_Blunders. Accessed 1 Apr 2016.
5. Time-management-guide.com. Essential goal setting guidelines. www.time-management-guide.com/goal-setting-guidelines.html. Accessed 1 Apr 2016.
6. Successful delegation, use the power of other people's help. https://www.mindtools.com/pages/article/newLDR_98.htm. Accessed 11 Mar 2016.

Selected Readings

Blanchard K, Johnson S. The one minute manager. New York: Berkeley Trade-William Morrow and Company, Inc.; 1982.

Connellan T. The 1% solution for work and life: how to make your next 30 days the best ever. Chelsea: Peak Performance Press, Inc; 2011.

Covey SR. The 7 habits of highly effective people. New York: Free Press – Simon & Schuster, Inc.; 2004.

The time management guide. http://www.time-management-guide.com/index.html. Last accessed 1 Apr 2016.

Wankat PC. The effective, efficient professor: teaching, scholarship, and service. Boston: Allyn & Bacon; 2002.

Index

A

Accreditation Council for Graduate Medical Education (ACGME), 21, 42, 97, 175
Adequate power, 26
Administrative data, 57, 58, 82, 84, 86, 87
Affordable Care Act, 83
Agency for Healthcare Quality and Research (AHRQ), 87, 102, 104
Alcohol abuse, 177
Alpha error. *See* Type I errors
The American College of Surgeons (ACS), 18, 21, 42, 57, 87, 97, 104, 105, 177, 181
American College of Surgeons National Surgical Quality Improvement Program (ACS-NSQIP), 57, 87
American College of Surgeons-National Surgical Quality Improvement Program (ACS-NSQIP), 57
American Healthcare System, 80
American Pediatric Surgical Association, 136, 177
Analysis of variance (ANOVA), 55
Anaplastic lymphoma kinase (ALK), 110
Animal models for surgical research
    large, 73–74
    murine
        clinical physiology, 74
        non-cancer models, 73–74
        phenotypic mimicry models, 74–75
        transgenic models, 69–70
        xenograft models, 70–73
    zebra fish, 75, 76
Anticipated/expected results, 29, 43, 155
Appropriate conclusions, 27

The Association for Academic Surgery (AAS), 18, 19, 21, 97, 101–105
Association for Surgical Education (ASE), 97, 101–105
The Association of American Medical Colleges (AAMC), 97, 103, 105
The Association of Program Directors in Surgery (APDS), 97, 102, 103, 105
Audiovideo (AV), operating room, 89
Authorship, 33, 41–42, 128–129, 142
Available population, 28

B

Bar chart, 56, 57, 123
Bariatric surgery, 7, 90, 91
Beta error. *See* Type II errors
Bias, 25–27, 29, 30, 34, 35, 40, 41, 44, 49–52, 58, 60–63
Bimodal distributions, 53, 54
Box plot, 55, 56
Bridge tenders, 3–4
Burnout, 176–179, 181–183

C

Career development awards (CDAs), 17–19
Case-control studies, 48, 49
Case reports/case-series, 48
Center for Medicare and Medicaid Services (CMS), 90
Chi-square tests, 57
Clinical and Translational Science Award (CTSA), 109
Clustering, 60, 63, 111
Cluster randomized trials, 80, 82

Cochran-Armitage trend test, 57
Cochran Q test, 57
Cohort studies, 48–49
The Common Rule, 36
Comparative effectiveness research (CER), 81–83
Compared with Research Project Grants (R awards), 145
Complimentary DNAs (cDNAs), 110, 111
Confirmation bias, 30
Conflict of interest, 30–41, 128
Confounder, 30, 49, 50, 58, 59, 61, 63–65, 82
Confounding, 26, 49, 50, 58, 61–66, 82, 92, 177
Confounding variables, 26
Consulting, with experts, 27
Coronary artery bypass graft (CABG), 87
Cross-sectional studies, 48
Curriculum vitae (CV), 9, 20

D
The Declaration of Helsinki, 36
Depression, 177, 178
Difference-in-difference analysis, 62, 63, 91, 92
Dishonesty, 43–44
Dissemination and implementation (D&I) reaearch, 88, 89
Donabedian model, 85
Dot plots, 55
Dual loyalties, surgeon-scientist, 34–35

E
Early retirement, 178
Effect size, 30
Electrospray ionization and mass spectroscopy (ESI-MS), 113
Eligible population, 28
e-mentoring, 137
Empirical Bayes techniques, 87
Errors, in medical research, 49–50
Ethical Principles for Medical Research Involving Human Subjects, 36
Ethics
    authorship, 41–42
    concerns, 33
    conflict of interest, 40–41
    dishonesty
        fabrication, 43
        falsification, 43
        plagiarism, 43–44
    human subject research
        The Common Rule, 36
        The Declaration of Helsinki, 36
        ethical requirements, 36–38

IRB, 36
Jewish chronic disease hospital, 36
Nuremberg code, 36
Tuskegee Syphilis studies, 36
World War II, 35
informed consent, 38–39
innovation *versus* research, 40
open research environment, 44
publication, 41–42
quality improvement, 42–43
surgeon-scientist dual loyalties, 34–35
triple-checking, 44
Ewing's sarcoma cells, 71, 72
Exogenous gene, 69
Experimental studies, 48, 49
Experiments and Observations of the Gastric Juice and the Physiology of Digestion, 34
Expert consultation, 27, 30
Externally valid study, 26, 27

F
False discovery rate (FDR), 111
Federal Coordinating Council, 81
Fisher exact test, 57
Forced expiratory volume (FEV1), 59

G
Gene-expression profiling, 110–112
Genomics, 109–110
Grant writing/writers
    avoiding common mistakes, 157–159
    candidate
        addressing limitations, 151–152
        past experiences, 151
        publication record, 151
        successful applicants, 150
    career development plan
        academic deficiencies, 152
        application process, 157
        clinical work and research balance, 153
        degree program, 152–153
        importance, 152
        mentor-mentee relationship, 153
        organizational and formatting tips, 156
    K awards and R awards comparison, 145
    mentor selection, 148–149
    NIH, 146–148
    research plan
        FoMO (Fear of Missing Out), 154
        narration, 156
        preliminary data, 154
        RePORT, 154

secondary data proposals, 155
Specific Aims, 155
statistician, 156
study design, 155–156
Green fluorescent protein (GFP), 71

H
Health Affairs, 92
Health services research (HSR)
definition, 79
disease management evaluation
CER, 81–83
data synthesis, 84
PCOR, 83–84
domains, 80
healthcare delivery system
policy evaluation, 90–91
surgical workforce, 91–92
local system of care
disparities, 85–86
implementation science, 88–89
patient safety, 89–90
quality measurement, 86–88
research techniques, 81
Heat shock protein 27 (HSP27), 114
Hierarchical clustering, 111
Hierarchical modeling, 87
High-performance liquid chromatography (HPLC), 113
Histograms, 55, 56
Hospital discharge data, 57
HSR. *See* Health services research (HSR)
Human hepatocellular carcinoma (HCC), 112, 114
Human Metabolome Database, 115
Huntington's disease, 110
Hypothesis development
anticipated/expected results, 29
available population, 28
eligible population, 28
null hypothesis, 29
principal/primary question, 28
reference population, 28
relevant, 27–28
specific intervention, 29
study population, 28
Hypothesis testing, 50, 52

I
Impact factor, 4–5
Informal mentoring, 137
Information bias, 26

Informed consent, 33, 36–40, 108
Institutional review board (IRB), 36, 43, 88, 163
Instructions to Authors, 121–122
Instrumental variable (IV) analysis, 50, 61–65, 82, 92
Internally valid study, 26
International Classification of Diseases, Clinical Modification (ICD-CM)-9, 57
Interquartile range, 53, 55, 56
Interstitial fibrosis and tubular atrophy (IFTA), 112
Isobaric tags for relative and absolute quantitation (iTRAQ), 114

J
Jewish chronic disease hospital, 36
Joint Photographic Experts Group (JPEG), 122
Journal, choosing, 120–121
Journal of the American Medical Association (JAMA), 82, 85–87, 91, 121
Junior researcher, 41, 42

K
Kaplan-Meier analysis, 65
K awards, 18, 145–152, 155, 157
Kruskal-Wallis test, 55

L
Lead time bias, 26
Linear regression analysis, 58–59
Line chart/graph, 56, 57, 123
Literature review
adequate power, 26
alpha error/type I error, 27
appropriate conclusions, 27
confounding variables, 26
expert consultations, 27
externally valid study, 26, 27
information bias, 26
internally valid, 26
lead time bias, 26
Medline, 26
misclassification errors, 26
multiple sources, 25
publication bias, 27
selection bias, 26
time bias, 26
time lag bias, 27
Logistic regression analysis, 59
Luciferase, 71, 72
Luminex 100 xMAP system, 113

M

Making the Right Moves: A Practical Guide to Scientific management for Postdocs and New Faculty, 167
Mann–Whitney *U* test. *See* Wilcoxon rank sum test
Manuscript writing. *See* Writing manuscript
McNemar test, 57
Mean, 53–55, 88
MedEdPortal, 105
Median, 53–56, 88, 111, 178
Medical Subject Headings (MeSH), 26
The Medicare and Medicaid Act of 1965, 175
Medicare Payment Advisory Commission (MedPAC), 92
Medline, 26
Mentored Career Development Award Grants. *See* K awards
Mentored Clinical Scientist Research Career Development Award (K08), 17, 18, 145, 146
Mentored Patient-Oriented Research Career Development Award (K23), 17, 18, 145, 146
Mentor/mentoring
  barriers, 135
  choosing right, 138
  informal, 137
  key features of successful, 138, 139
  from mentee to colleague, 141
  mentor-candidate's track record, 140
  modern definition, 137
  multiple mentors, 140
  networking, 137–138
  origin, 136
  risks, 141–142
  selecting appropriate research, 148–149
  sponsorship, 137
  spontaneous/accidental, 137
  traditional functions, 137
  women and men, 135–136
Metabolomics, 115, 116
Misclassification errors, 26
MLM. *See* Multilevel modeling (MLM)
Mode, 53
Multilevel modeling (MLM), 60
Multivariable analysis, 58
Murine for surgical research
  clinical physiology, 74
  non-cancer models, 73–74
  phenotypic mimicry models, 74–75
  transgenic models, 69–70
  xenograft models, 70–73

N

The National Cancer Data Bank, 57
National Cancer Database, 87
National Cancer Institute (NCI), 108
National Center for Advancing Translational Sciences (NCATS), 108–109
National Heart, Lung, and Blood Institute's (NHLBI), 147
National Initiative for Cancer Care Quality, 85
National Institutes of Health (NIH), 10, 11, 13, 17, 18, 21, 69, 83, 102, 107–109, 130, 136, 145–148, 150, 154, 157–159
National Medicare data, 87, 91
National Patient Safety Foundation, 89
National Research Service Award (NRSA), 10, 11
National Trauma Database, 87
Nationwide Inpatient Sample (NIS), 57, 87
Necrotizing enterocolitis (NEC), 74
New England Journal of Medicine, 85, 88
Non-cancer models, 73–74
Non-small cell lung cancer (NSCLC), 110
Null hypothesis, 29, 50
Nuremberg code, 36
Nuremberg trials, 36

O

Observational studies, 47–50, 57–58, 61, 62
  case-control studies, 48, 49
  case reports/case-series, 48
  cohort studies, 48–49
  cross-sectional studies, 48
  EUS, 65–66
  IOC and common duct injury, 62–65
Office for Human Research Protection (OHRP), 88
Oncogene, 69, 70
Open research environment, 44
Orthotopic xenograft models, 71
Outcome reporting bias, 30

P

Patient-centered outcomes research (PCOR), 81, 83–84
Patient safety, 6, 7, 80, 89–90, 102
Pearson's correlation, 111
Percentiles, 55
Phosphoglycerate mutase 1 (PGAM1), 114
Plagiarism, 43
Policy evaluation, 90–91

Polymerase chain reaction (PCR), 111
Power analysis, 29
Pragmatic clinical trials, 80, 82
Premier Hospital Incentive Demonstration, 91
Principal/primary question, 28
Professional societies, surgical education, 105
Promotion timeline
   approaching promotion, 19–20
   assistant professor, 12–13
      job search, 12–13
      transition to full professor, 20–21
   CDAs, 17–19
   definition, 9
   first three years
      potential tracks, 14
      surgical journals, 15
      T&P process, 16
   mid-career move, 19
   preparation phase, 10–11
Propensity score (PS) analysis, 61, 64–66, 82
Proteomics, 112–115
Publication bias, 27
P-value, 27, 50, 52, 55, 57, 59, 125

Q

Quintessential animal model, 69

R

Randomized controlled trials, 30
Rat insulin promoter (RIP), 70
R awards, 145, 146, 152
Reference population, 28
Research integrity, 30
Research Portfolio Online Reporting Tools (RePORT) system, 154
R01 grant, 11, 107, 148, 155
Rip-tag model, 69
Robotic technology, 40

S

Scatter plots, 55
Science research program
   advertising, 166
   conducting structured interview, 167
   decisions, 162
   hiring process, 165–166
   interviews
   laboratory personnel, 164–165
   mission/vision, 162–163
   planning projects, 163
   probation period, 167
   program leadership, 170–171
   references, 166–167
   research techniques, 170
   saving money, 163–164
   seeking help, 164
   time management, 169–170
   trainees
      duration, 169
      funding, 169
      postdoctoral, 168
      primary role, 167–168
      surgeon-scientist, 168
      writing skills, 168
Secondary data analysis, 57–58
Secondary questions, 28
SEER. *See* Surveillance Epidemiology and End Results (SEER)
Selection bias, 26
   difference-in-difference analysis, 62, 63
   IV analysis, 61–62
   MLM, 60
   PS analysis, 61
Sepsis, 74, 112
Significance Analysis of Microarrays (SAM), 111
Simian Virus 40 (SV40), 69, 70
Single nucleotide polymorphism (SNP), 109
The Society of University Surgeons, 40, 97, 105, 169
Society of University Surgeons (SUS), 97
Spearman's correlation, 111
Sponsorship, 137
Spontaneous/accidental mentoring, 137
Standard deviation (SD), 30, 53, 55, 111
Statistical analysis
   categorical variables comparison, 56–57
   central tendency
      mean, 53, 54
      median, 53, 54
      mode, 53, 54
   linear regression analysis, 58–59
   logistic regression analysis, 59
   measure of spread
      interquartile range, 53, 55, 56
      percentiles, 55
      range, 54
      standard deviation, 55
   multivariable analysis, 58
   numeric variables comparison, 55
   time-to-event analyses, 59–60
Statistical inferences
   power, 52

P-value, 50, 52
type I errors, 50, 52
type II error, 52
Stem-and-leaf plots, 55
Study design
  confirmation bias, 30
  effect size, 30
  experimental studies, 48, 49
  expert consultations, 30–31
  observational studies
    case-control studies, 48, 49
    case reports/case-series, 48
    cohort studies, 48–49
    cross-sectional studies, 48
  outcome reporting bias, 30
  power analysis, 29
  randomized controlled trials, 30
  research integrity, 30
Study population, 28
Suicide, 177, 178
Surgical Care Improvement Program (SCIP), 86, 87
Surgical educational research
  assessment, 100
  benefits, 96
    accomplishment/gratification, 97–98
    career advancement opportunities, 97
    challenges, 96
    low barrier to entry, 96
    opportunity for national involvement, 97
  challenges, 96
    academic credibility, 98
    limited funding, 98
    limited mentorship, 98
    limited statistical power, 98
  starting
    forums for publication/presentation, 103, 105
    funding opportunities, 102–104
    surgical education research team, 101–102
  topics
    curriculum and teaching, 100
    simulation, 99–100
    team training, 100–101
Surgical innovation, 39–40, 102, 155, 157
SURgical PAtient Safety System (SURPASS), 88
Surgical research
  basic science research, 6
  clinical studies, 6
  outcomes research/HSR, 6–7
  surgical education research, 7
  translational research, 6
Surgical residents, 15, 98, 100, 175
Surveillance Epidemiology and End Results (SEER), 57, 65, 82

T

Tagged Image File Format (TIFF), 122
T antigen transgene (TAg), 70
Time bias, 26, 30, 51
Time lag bias, 27
Time management
  assessment, 188
  buffer time, 193
  definition, 187
  delegation
    action plans, 190–191
    activity logs, 191
    urgency-importance matrix, 189–190
  goal setting
    completing large tasks, 194–196
    SMART concept, 194, 196
    tips, 195
  maximizing efficiency
    getting organized, 196
    improving daily efficiency, 197
    multitasking, 197
    postive thoughts, 198
    tips, 197
    work life balance, 198
  planning and prioritizing, 189
  saying "no," 189–191
  scheduling protected time
    buffer time, 193
    eliminating distractions, 193
    email, 194, 195
    time savers, 192
    time wasters, 192
  strategies, 188
  to-do list, 189
Time-to-event analyses, 59–60
Title 45 CFR 46. *See* The Common Rule
T&P process, 16
Transgenic models, 69–70
Translational research, 6, 10, 14, 17, 18, 33, 96, 107–116, 161
Translational Research Working Group (TRWG), 108
Traumatic brain injury (TBI), 115
t test, 55, 111
Tumor registries, 57
Tuskegee Syphilis studies, 36
Type I errors, 27, 50, 52
Type II errors, 26, 52

U

United States Department of Health and Human Services, 36
Univariate analysis, 55
Urgency-importance matrix, 189–190

V

Variables
  categorical
    nominal data, 53
    ordinal data, 53
  numerical data
    continuous scale, 53
    discrete scale, 53
Vertebrate models, 75–76
Virtual mentoring, 137

W

Wilcoxon rank sum test, 55
Work-life imbalance
  adverse consequences
    burn out, 176–179, 181–183
    magnitude of the problem, 176–177
    personal level, 177–178
    professional level, 178
  change, in surgical culture, 183
  generation Y, 176
  millennials, 176
  prevention and recovery
    personal level, 179–181
    professional level, 181–182
  surgical residents, 175
World Medical Association, 36
Writing manuscript
  abstract, 128
  acknowledgments, 127–128
  authorship, 128–129
  discussion, 126–127
  figure legends, 125
  figures, 123
  importance, 119–120
  instructions to authors, 121–122
  introduction, 125–126
  journal choosing, 120–121
  manuscript writing order, 122–123
  methods, 124
  order, 122–123
  place of, 120
  responding to reviewer comments, 131
  results, 124–125
  revising before submission, 129–130
  rules of academic, 120
  successful award application, 150
  tables, 123
  timing, 120
  title, 128

X

Xenograft models, 70–73

Z

Zebrafish, 75, 76

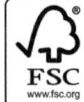

MIX
Papier aus verantwortungsvollen Quellen
Paper from responsible sources
FSC® C105338

If you have any concerns about our products,
you can contact us on
ProductSafety@springernature.com

In case Publisher is established outside the EU,
the EU authorized representative is:
**Springer Nature Customer Service Center GmbH
Europaplatz 3, 69115 Heidelberg, Germany**

Printed by Libri Plureos GmbH
in Hamburg, Germany